DATE DUE

Unde
Beha a
that

A Guide nent

Ian And

Jessica Kingsley *Publishers*
London and Philadelphia

First published in 2011
by Jessica Kingsley Publishers
116 Pentonville Road
London N1 9JB, UK
and
400 Market Street, Suite 400
Philadelphia, PA 19106, USA

www.jkp.com

Library of Congress Cataloging in Publication Data
A CIP catalog record for this book is available from the Library of Congress

British Library Cataloguing in Publication Data
A CIP catalogue record for this book is available from the British Library

ISBN 978 1 84905 108 8

Printed and bound in Great Britain

Contents

Figures

Tables

Introduction

THE RISING PROFILE OF DEMENTIA

In recent years the topic of dementia has received a lot of attention internationally (Vernooij-Dassen *et al.* 2010). In 2010, the *International Journal of Geriatric Psychiatry* dedicated a special issue on the global response with respect to the management of dementia (Burns 2010). In the UK, all of the four home countries are publishing, or have already published, national dementia strategies and plans (England, Scotland, Wales and Northern Ireland). Throughout the world governments are preparing for the consequences of ageing populations and the tsunami of dementia related issues. This is in marked contrast to the whole of the previous century in which this condition received comparatively little attention at a governmental level in relation to conditions such as cancer and heart disease. The Health Economic Research Centre, UK (HERC 2010) calculated that Government and charitable spending on dementia research is 12 times lower than on cancer research (£50 million compared to £590 million), and less than a third of the spending on heart disease (£169 million). This is in contrast to the cost of the three diseases to the economy, with dementia costing £23 billion, cancer £12 billion and heart disease £8 billion.

The major spurs in the UK have been key publications such as the National Audit Office's 'Improving Services and Support for People with Dementia' (NAO 2007); 'Remember, I'm still me' (CC/MWC 2009) and the National Dementia Strategies for England (DoH 2009) and Scotland (Scottish Government 2010). Many of the influential documents have been critical of existing service provision. For example, The Audit Commission's publication of 'Forget Me Not' (CHAI 2002) was critical of the role of professionals, particularly primary care services, and 'Living Well in Later Life' (2006) described the problems in attempting to implement the National Service Framework for Older People (DoH 2001).

To illustrate some of the reasons for the UK government's concerns consider the following data and demographics (information from NAO 2007; DoH, National Dementia Strategy for England 2009b; Time for Action report, Banerjee 2009; HERC 2010):

- 820,000 people in the UK have dementia; this is 1.3 per cent of the population. The majority of these people live in England.

- Approximately 30 per cent of people (230,000) with dementia in the UK live in care homes.

- 15,000 people with dementia are under 65 years of age, and services for this younger group are underdeveloped.

- 15,000 dementia sufferers come from minority ethnic groups, and this figure is set to rise sharply owing to the ageing of people who settled in the UK from the 1950s onwards.

- 69 per cent of General Practitioners (GPs) do not believe they have received sufficient training to diagnose dementia and manage difficult behaviours. This is a decrease in perceived abilities compared to 8 years ago ('Forget Me Not' report 2002), and may be accounted for by the increasing expectation from service-users and their families.

- 25 per cent of people with dementia in the UK are prescribed anti-psychotics, mainly for the treatment of problematic behaviours. These drugs have significant side-effects, and are effective in only one in five presentations.

- The national cost of dementia per year is £23 billion (50% for the cost of unpaid care; 40% social care costs; 10% health care costs).

The English National Dementia Strategy was launched in 2009, and was promised £150 million to oversee its implementation. Within the 17 objectives of the strategy, we see a positive vision of what good care provision could look like. However, few of the objectives specifically address behaviours that challenge (BCs), which are major sources of carer and family distress, and the reason why many people require hospitalisation or 24-hour care. The Scottish strategy provides more guidance on BCs, overtly articulating issues to do with client distress and the need for staff training. The current book intends to expand on many of the points made in these strategies, focusing on the perspectives of clinicians working with clients who are deemed to be challenging.

BEHAVIOURS THAT CHALLENGE (BC)

Behaviours that challenge were previously referred to as challenging behaviours. The latter term originally came from the learning disability literature and was used to describe problematic behaviours that cause difficulties for the person performing them, or for the setting in which they are displayed. Blunden and Allen (1987) suggest the term was introduced in order to shift the focus of attention away from individual pathology towards an understanding that challenges carers and service providers to find solutions to the problem behaviours. Many old age psychiatrists prefer to use the term behavioural and psychological symptoms of dementia (BPSD) to denote the link to dementia in their work. However, the term BPSD has been criticised because it implies the problematic behaviours are linked directly to the dementing process. As we will see in Chapter 1, this is clearly not the case because many of the behaviours are normal coping strategies used by the general population to deal with difficult settings.

This book contains eight chapters, providing theory and practical advice on the treatment of BC, using a biopsychosocial perspective. Thus it suggests that the management of BC should take account of the combined influences of the chemical neurological, physical changes, as well as the psychological and social features. In each of the following chapters this perspective will be illustrated and expanded upon, using case examples and research data. For example, Chapter 1 will examine the concept of BC, providing an overview of types of behaviours and categorisation systems. Chapter 2 examines the common causes of BCs, and provides examples of assessment tools. Chapters 3 and 4 describe the current treatment strategies, discussing the pharmacological and non-pharmacological approaches. Both of these approaches have been criticised because of their poor evidence bases, with particular concerns about the problematic side-effects of medication. Chapter 5 outlines a number of different conceptual models that have been developed in the field to enhance people's understanding of dementia and BCs. By gaining better awareness, it is suggested that clinicians' assessments and treatment strategies may be improved.

In the later chapters of the book, there will be a greater focus on practice and service issues. Chapter 6 describes the clinical approach I have developed with colleagues in Newcastle for working into 24-hour care settings. In Chapter 7 a number of case examples are presented, with comprehensive descriptions of the treatment processes.

Chapter 8 addresses the issue of service development, drawing on the recent government commissioned report 'Time for Action' (Banerjee 2009). In this report, that was accepted by the Minister of State, its author calls for a radical overhaul of BC services and treatment approaches; with a move from an anti-psychotic dominated mode of treatment to one that makes better use of non-pharmacological approaches. Indeed, Banerjee calls for a reduction in anti-psychotic usage of two-thirds over a three-year period, and puts forward 11 recommendations to allow this to be achieved.

RELEVANCE OF THIS BOOK

This book is timely as we start to implement the recommendations of the various national strategies. It is also relevant because there remains a great deal of confusion regarding the treatment of BC. Many psychiatrists think that they have been put in a difficult situation regarding the proposed restrictions on the use of medications, particularly the use of anti-psychotics. It is relevant to note, however, that psychiatrists continue to have a lot of faith in these drugs and are still prescribing them on a regular basis (Wood-Mitchell et al. 2008; Bishara et al. 2009). Currently, non-medical professionals may also be at a loss, because they have received little 'quality' guidance on what to offer as a practical alternative to drugs. Indeed, many of the non-pharmacological strategies suggested in the literature are preventative methods rather than treatment approaches. This book explores the distinction between 'prevention' and 'treatment' strategies and provides advice for dealing with BCs in their acute phases. This text also has particular relevance for those working in the private sector, describing a treatment approach designed to specifically work with residents in 24-hour care.

The book is also relevant to commissioners and government employees, particularly in light of the recent HERC (2010) publication that revealed each dementia client costs the UK economy £27,647 per year (cancer: £5999; heart disease: £3455). This figure does not include extra costs that are incurred when a client displays problematic behaviours.

It is evident that there is a need, and a desire, to improve care practices. The move away from a medical approach to BC is not new, it has been slowly happening over the last 20 years. However, the call for change has increased of late, gaining momentum owing to concerns about the use of drugs and the need to develop effective alternatives to them. In addition, and perhaps most importantly, additional impetus for change has come from our politicians and economists who seem to recognise that it is essential to plan for the future from both a financial and well-being perspective.

Chapter 1

Introduction to Behaviours that Challenge

DEFINITION

For the purposes of this book, behaviours that challenge (BC) are defined as actions that detract from the well-being of individuals due to the physical or psychological distress they cause within the settings they are performed. The individuals affected may be either the instigators of the acts or those in the immediate surroundings. Common BCs include: hitting, screaming, excessive pacing, apathy, etc. The BCs often have multiple causes (e.g. physical, mental, environmental, neurological), which are moderated by people's emotions and beliefs. BCs are common, and generally managed well by carers, and many resolve with time. However, some problems can become chronic or risky, and on these occasions specialist assistance is required in the form of biopsychosocial approaches (i.e. medical and non-pharmacological). Such approaches require a thorough assessment of the situation, and then effective targeting of the causal factors underlying the behaviours.

The definition will be unpacked in the remainder of this chapter, and the following aspects emphasised:

- BC are problematic behaviours that cause difficulties for the person performing them, or for the setting in which they are displayed.

- What is perceived to be 'challenging' will differ between settings, with some onlookers being more tolerant than others. For this reason, the term 'BC' is viewed as a 'social construct'.

- They often reflect some form of need that is either driven by a belief (e.g. the person thinks she needs to collect her children from school) or is related to distress (e.g. signalling or coping with discomfort/boredom).

- BCs have multiple causes, and the neurological impairment associated with dementia is just one of the numerous factors.

- Categorisation systems have been developed in order to group similar forms of behaviour into meaningful units. These groupings have formed the basis of treatment strategies.

- Owing to the complexities involved in treating chronic BCs, treatment protocols are useful management guides. The protocol developed by the Newcastle Challenging Behaviour Team (NCBT, i.e. the team I lead) is presented as an illustration.

NATURE OF BC

Cohen-Mansfield (2001) suggests that BC in dementia often reflect an attempt by a person to signal a need that is currently not being met (e.g. to indicate hunger; to gain relief from pain or boredom, etc.), or an effort by an individual to get his needs met directly (e.g. leave a building when he believes he must go to work or collect children from school), or as a sign of frustration (e.g. feeling angry at being told he is not allowed to exit a building). In all of these situations, the actions are attempts by the individual to enhance and maintain his sense of well-being or ease distress.

Behaviours are labelled as challenging when they are perceived to be negative in some way for either the perpetrator, or those impacted on by the actions. Indeed, in some circumstances the actor may be unaware that his actions are troublesome. For example, a person's habit of urinating in the corridor may be more problematic for his carers than for him. For an action to be perceived as challenging a threshold needs to be passed, and this requires a judgement by a carer. As the judgements tend to be determined by the tolerance of carers and care settings, the term BC is often applied inconsistently. Indeed, what is acceptable in one environment may be seen as intolerable by carers in a different setting. Hence, the phenomenon of BC is seen as a social construct rather than a true clinical disorder that can be reliably measured.

A comprehensive list of BC is provided in Table 1.1. As one can see, BC are not specific to dementia, rather they are actions frequently observed in the general population. Indeed, many of these acts are common occurrences outside many UK pubs and bars most weekend evenings.

Table 1.1 List of common behaviours that challenge (BCs)

Aggressive forms of BCs	Non-aggressive forms of BCs
Hitting	Apathy
Kicking	Depression
Grabbing	Repetitive noise
Pushing	Repetitive questions
Nipping	Making strange noises
Scratching	Constant requests for help
Biting	Eating/drinking excessively
Spitting	Over-activity
Choking	Pacing
Hair pulling	General agitation
Tripping someone	Following others/trailing
Throwing objects	Inappropriate exposure of parts of body
Stick prodding	
Stabbing	Masturbating in public areas
Swearing	Urinating in inappropriate places
Screaming	Smearing
Shouting	Handling things inappropriately
Physical sexual assault	Dismantling objects
Verbal sexual advances	Hoarding things
Acts of self-harm	Hiding items
	Falling intentionally
	Eating inappropriate substances
	Non-compliance
	Misidentifying

It is worth noting that there are many difficulties associated with defining BC in terms of behaviours. This is in part because it encourages clinicians to think of people's difficulties in terms of their outwards signs (i.e. the actions) rather than their underlying cause(s). For example, by labelling a BC as 'aggression', one might be distracted from identifying its true cause which might be either pain or paranoia. Figure 1.1 is a diagram that serves to remind us about the links between behaviours and their causes.

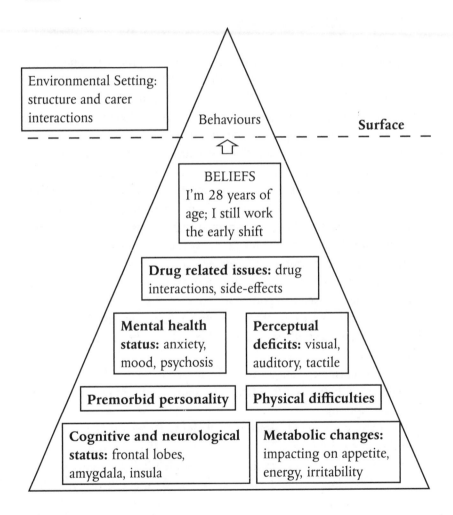

Figure 1.1 BC iceberg analogy

As can be seen from the diagram, the link between the behaviours and their causes is often via some form of belief. Such beliefs are often emotionally charged by fear, anger, pride or despair. The beliefs are also related to 'needs', whereby a person who believes he is still working, may have a perceived need to leave the building at 5 am to do his morning shift. The causes, and their interactions with each other, will be explored further in the next chapter.

CATEGORISATION OF BCS

Over the last ten years researchers have tried to identify different categories of BC. Cohen-Mansfield 2000b has produced one of the most valid and helpful ways of differentiating between them; she distinguishes between physically aggressive acts (hitting, hair pulling); physically non-aggressive (pacing, over-activity) and verbally disruptive behaviours (shouting, repetitive questioning).

Based on these categories, Cohen-Mansfield has provided a useful framework for helping to determine causes of BCs, termed TREA (Treatment Routes for Exploring Agitation, Coleen-Mansfield 2000b). TREA is a comprehensive approach designed to help staff to identify causes and corresponding treatment plans. It uses a decision tree questionnaire format in which one arrives at the most likely cause of a problematic behaviour by assessment of the category and type of behaviour, the setting, and information about the individual (see Table 1.2). Once a cause has been hypothesised, one of a selection of treatments is chosen and carried out. If that treatment is unsuccessful, another is chosen, or a new hypothesis generated based on a better understanding of the problem.

Cohen-Mansfield's questions differ for each of her three categories of challenging behaviour (physical non-aggression, physical aggression, verbal disruption).

For many years the Newcastle Challenging Behaviour Team (NCBT) used the above categorisation system to good effect. However, recently we have become interested in the role of people's belief systems as causal features of BC (see Figure 1.1). As such, and from audits of our clinical work, we developed an alternate categorisation system (see Table 1.3). This system distinguishes between non-active and active forms of BC. The non-active types are related to apathy and depression. These are the most common categories of BC (Renauld *et al.* 2010; Moniz-Cook *et al.*

2001b). Some clinicians may not regard these behaviours as challenging, but clearly the conditions are distressing for the individuals experiencing them, and certainly undermine their levels of well-being.

Table 1.2 Some questions to be used in the case of physical non-aggressive behaviours

Question 1	Question 2	Potential treatment
Does the person seem upset?	Is the person asking for home?	Try to make the place look more like home
	Is the person restless?	Try to find activities which are meaningful
	Is the person uncomfortable?	Change position or provide other sources of comfort
Does the person have a need for self-stimulation or exercise?	Are you concerned about the safety of the person?	Try to use safety devices: safety alarms, large enclosed environments, change appearance of exit door
	Is the person trespassing and bothering others?	Try to develop a more inviting environment where the person can wander, camouflage other entrances

In relation to the active forms of BC, we have distinguished four types. The first group can be conceptualised as reactions to stressful situations. In this group, people can feel vulnerable, think their rights are being infringed, or feel frustrated that they are not being listened to. The BCs may be caused by misinterpretations of situations due to perceptual problems, or memory deficits or psychotic features (hallucinations or delusions). Thus their reactions to these perceptions are to either seek reassurance or become aggressive.

The second group of active BC are typified by walking and interfering activities. These behaviours reflect attempts by the clients to orientate themselves to their surroundings, which may be difficult due to their cognitive and memory problems.

Third, there is a group of BC that result from failures by the person with dementia to inhibit actions, thoughts and emotions. This group of behaviours is closely related to frontal lobe deficits.

Finally, there are behaviours that reflect a mismatch between the person and the environment he is in. These disruptive behaviours stem from the person rejecting the setting. For example, the person may not like the restrictions or features of his current living conditions. These various categories of BC are summarised in Table 1.3. We have found the distinctions useful, for despite some overlaps within groups, they help distinguish behaviours on social, neurological and emotional grounds, thus helping clinicians to see the sorts of things that might be driving the behaviours. And consequently, the groups provide some theoretical guidance towards treatment strategies.

The NCBT categorisation system differs in a number of ways to Cohen-Mansfield's, but one of the chief differences is that it does not categorise by an actions typology, rather it focuses more on the causal features (i.e. the features driving the behaviour). Hence, a behaviour such as 'excessive walking' could be placed within a number of categories – it could be due to a disinhibition, anxiety, or an attempt to find a way out of the building. Recognising which category it belongs within the NCBT framework helps one to direct one's intervention.

MANAGING BCs: A TREATMENT PROTOCOL

BC are common in dementia, with 90 per cent of those with dementia displaying some form of BC during their illness (Lyketsos *et al.* 2002). They often occur in the later stages of the illness, and there is an association with severity of BC and severity of dementia (Thompson *et al.* 2010). In most circumstances they are dealt with well by carers, with few problematic consequences. However, occasionally the behaviours persist, and some may even be reinforced by carers' actions. It is in these latter circumstances that specialist help may be required either in the form of medication or non-pharmacological approaches.

Table 1.3 BC categories derived from an audit of NCBT clinical work

Type of BC	Emotions and beliefs	Comment
Lack of motivation and initiation (non-active form of BC)	Apathy or depression associated with beliefs of helplessness and worthlessness.	Behaviourally apathy and depression look similar, but apathy is related to brain changes in the frontal lobes. In contrast depression is often a consequence of the person's poor sense of worth and sense of hopelessness. Referrals for amotivation are common from family carers, but uncommon for residents in care homes. This is because care staff find it easier to look after residents who are less active; thus the behaviour is often not seen as problematic in the context of the setting.
Threat related (active form of BC)	Anxiety and anger – on occasions anxiety precedes anger, with the anger being the active response when feeling threatened. Anxiety is associated with beliefs of being vulnerable. Anger is related to a sense that one's rights are being infringed and one is being treated unjustly.	The actions are responses to emotional experiences, whether related to interactions with others or psychotic hallucinations or delusions. The person may feel fearful or threatened and thus avoid situations, or seek safety. On other occasions the person might react to a perceived threat with aggression either as a defence or as a pre-emptive action. Sometimes the threat is related to the person's self-esteem, and the response is due to a self-perception that her rights are being infringed (James 2001). From a neurological perspective, damage to the amygdala or right somatosensory cortex (RSc) is associated with anger and anxiety. The amygdala processes emotions and is closely linked to the frontal lobes. The RSc is involved in the processing of people's body language and emotional expressions. Thus problems here can lead to misinterpretation of other people's intentions.

Table 1.3 BC categories derived from an audit of NCBT clinical work *cont.*

Type of BC	Emotions and beliefs	Comment
Information and solution seeking (active)	Curiosity and problem-solving behaviours – natural engagement with one's surroundings, disrupted by memory problems, confusion, disorientation, and boredom. Associated with a belief that one must seek someone or something out to make sense of the situation.	Humans are natural explorers and problem solvers. When a person feels disorientated or confused she will attempt to reduce these uncomfortable states by either asking about, or exploring, her surroundings. Likewise if she comes across an object that is in some way familiar or interesting (perhaps relating to work or home-life) she may borrow it, use it or even try to dismantle it.
Failure to inhibit (active)	Sexual disinhibition, repetitive vocalisations and repetitive actions. Associated with egocentric beliefs and thoughts which are often impulsive.	Reduced frontal lobe functioning is one of the few universal features of an ageing brain (Schaie 2008). However, for some people this can result in them having difficulties in inhibiting inappropriate actions and speech (aka thought-action fusion – impulsively doing or saying what you think).
Poor environmental fit (active)	Rejection of one's surrounding. Associated with beliefs about leaving the unpleasant setting.	The rejection may be due to a failure to recognise one's surrounding or the people in it, or due to the perceived restraints imposed by the settings (i.e. the rules, regulations and attempts to control one's life).

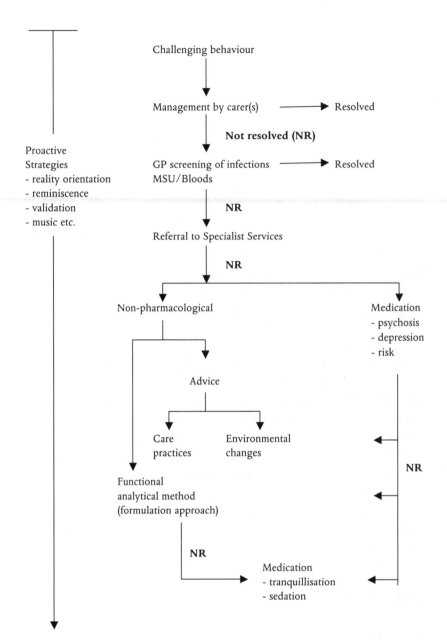

Figure 1.2 BC management protocol

A diagrammatic representation of a BC management protocol is provided in Figure 1.2. It identifies the various incremental steps used to treat problematic behaviours. The first step is the labelling of a behaviour as a 'challenge', followed by the initial attempts to resolve the difficulty by the carers. If the problems persist, an acute physical cause may be suspected, requiring an assessment from the primary care practitioner (e.g. a GP). If the GP fails to identify any infection on screening, she may suggest the referral to a specialist mental health service. At this point there are three possible responses, one pharmacological and two non-pharmacological. In terms of the former, if a discrete clinical disorder is identified (psychosis, depression, pain, delirium), then it will be treated through the use of medication. Or, if the behaviour is so extreme or risky, the appropriate medication may be given to tranquillise or sedate the person with dementia on a short-term basis. In relation to psychological approaches, one may either offer advice after undertaking a cursory assessment, or undertake a full functional analytical (FA, Moniz-Cook *et al.* in press) treatment package. The latter approach is the most comprehensive, involving a thorough assessment and the use of behavioural charts. If the FA methodology is unsuccessful and the behaviour persists, one may treat the BC chiefly via medication, but at this stage the rationale for using the medication is as a tranquilliser or sedative in order to improve the client's well-being. Despite presenting this protocol in terms of sequential steps, it is relevant to note that many specialist services employ combined modes of treatment, using both non-pharmacological and drugs concurrently (Holmes 2009). It is my view that, owing to both the lack of efficacy and side-effects of the psychotropics used in this area, it is unethical to prescribe a drug without simultaneously prescribing a non-pharmacological strategy. Alistair Burns, UK National Clinical Director of Dementia, is currently working to produce a national set of treatment guidelines for BC.

CONCLUSION

This chapter has provided a brief introduction to some key topics which will be discussed in-depth in the later sections of the book. Because BC are not diagnosable disorders, with regular and consistent underlying causes, they will always be somewhat problematic to treat. Indeed, the method of treating them appropriately will invariably require one becoming a detective and gaining detailed information about the nature of the BC and the client. The kind of detail required and how to put it together into a coherent formulation-led treatment package is the subject of this book.

Chapter 2

Causes and Assessments

INTRODUCTION

This chapter examines some of the causes of BC and the variables associated with them. Details about these features are important, because they help clinicians develop effective treatments.

The key points emphasised in this chapter are:

- BCs often have a number of interacting biopsychosocial causes.

- It is important to identify the potential causes of BC because this helps with the development of targetted interventions.

- Clients' beliefs play an important role in the development and manifestation of their BC. Indeed, attempts by a person to act on his beliefs can result in problems (e.g. an 80-year-old man who believes he is 30, and still doing early shift-work, may have a strong motivation to leave the building early each morning).

- There are many measures that can be used in the assessment of the causes of BC. The majority are too lengthy to be used clinically, and tend to be employed in research settings.

BACKGROUND INFORMATION

As outlined in the previous chapter, the most comprehensive BC model to date has been developed by Cohen-Mansfield (2000a). Her TREA framework first identifies categories of behaviour, and asks relevant questions, leading to potential solutions. (e.g. Continually screaming → Does this happen when she is been transferred from wheel-chair to a bed/toilet? → If yes, attempt pain relief). This approach is also supported by her unmet needs model, which requires clinicians to undertake a detailed analysis of the behaviour as well as background details of the person and his environment. She suggests that obtaining this contextual information is often helpful in determining the causes of the BC (see Chapter 5). Consistent with this are the requirements of the NCBT framework, which asks clinicians to collect eight pieces of background information about the client. It is relevant to note that these are the aspects previously outlined in the Iceberg Model (see Figure 1.1). These features are discussed below in terms of three groupings: biological, psychological and social factors. In Chapter 7 a series of case studies illustrates how the information is used clinically.

Biological
Cognitive and neurological difficulties
The brain and its functions determine how a person sees and interprets his environment. In the case of dementia, the cognitive deficits will often mean the person has a different sense of reality to other people. For example, he may be disorientated in time and place, and may not remember what happened a few minutes earlier.

It is important to note that having a different view of the world to the people one is interacting with does not automatically make someone's behaviour challenging. However, it can bring the person into conflict with others, particularly if there is a dispute about whose views are correct. Consider an 85-year-old woman in care who is angry at being prevented from leaving the setting when she is convinced her children need to be collected from school.

Drugs
Polypharmacy is a fact of life for many older people, with the average older person taking five or more different types of medication. While we are aware of the side-effects of much of the medication used, we are less certain of the effects of the interactions. This is somewhat of a concern when we already know some of the drugs commonly used are known to increase BC, such as: statins (agitation) and Parkinson's medication (hypersexuality). Furthermore, there are also major concerns about the tranquillising and sedating effects of many of the drugs used to routinely treat BC (Banerjee 2009).

Physical difficulties and metabolic changes

Dementia is an age-related illness, and many older people experience declining physical health and age-related illnesses (arthritis, backache, cancer, toothache, constipation and chiropody ailments). It is important to note that many BCs are related to pain and physical discomfort, which is often worsened during carer interactions (such as toileting, transfers and washing procedures). The body's organs also become less efficient with age, leading to a reduction in the body's ability to metabolise chemicals, including food and drugs.

Perceptual deficits

Age-related changes with respect to the five senses can trigger difficulties, as sensory loss may disorientate people further. Reductions in sight and hearing may also cause people to seek reassurance, or motivate them to search their environment in order to gain their bearings. Hearing problems are often associated with shouting (Cohen-Mansfield 2000a).

Psychological
Premorbid personality

It is important to recognise that a person's personality endures through the course of dementia; their individuality will be apparent in various ways and at different stages of the illness. People with severe dementia may still wish to express lifestyle preferences (relating, for example, to accommodation, religious practices, food and sexual orientation). While some personality changes are related to changes in brain pathology, others are associated with psychological factors – for example, someone with dementia may feel they are vulnerable, become more emotional and seek out more physical attention. Finding out how the person coped with difficulties in the past can be revealing. Current problems may be explained by someone being unable to use familiar methods of coping, such as managing stress by going out for a walk.

Mental health

Mental health problems are common and it is important to acknowledge their potential influence. Past difficulties may interact with current problems; for example, a person with long-standing social phobic tendencies who develops dementia and moves into residential care may feel very anxious in a busy communal room (James and Sabin 2002).

Changes in brain pathology may result in psychotic symptoms such as visual hallucinations, paranoid ideations or delusions of theft. Resolved issues, such as affective problems, may re-emerge, and chronic problems become magnified (e.g. Asperger traits, James *et al.* 2006c).

Social
Environment and care practice

Environmental factors (light, noise levels, room-layout) are important influences on the well-being of older people owing to their levels of dependency. This is particularly the case for people with dementia who have difficulties with memory, problem-solving and orientation. We need to recognise the link between people's level of well-being and the opportunities they have to engage in fulfilling personal relationships. It is also worth checking whether a person's 'challenging behaviour' might be triggered by him being too hot, too cold, hungry or being exposed to excessive stimulation such as a loud television or radio (DSDC 2008).

Care practices

Owing to the need for people with dementia to receive various forms of physical and practical help with aspects of daily living, conflict may arise with those providing such assistance. Carers are required to be skilled, patient practitioners and to have excellent communication skills. Such an angelic demeanour is not always possible, especially when there are competing issues with respect to carers' time. As such, in many BC situations the triggers for the problems can be traced to carers outpacing the person with dementia, being too rushed or abrupt, and unempathic. The relevance of good care practices cannot be over-emphasised because many challenging behaviours occur during practical face-to-face interactions between carers and clients.

The biopsychosocial factors presented above are believed to be common causes of problematic behaviours. Hence, when investigating the potential causes of a BC, one would routinely collect information about each of the above aspects. The next section presents tables outlining causal features for BC, resulting from an audit undertaken of the case work of a member of the NCBT (Makin 2009).

Table 2.1 The common biopsychosocial causes of shouting

Shouting – one needs to distinguish the various forms of shouting – shrieks, moans, repetitive words or sentences. Also one needs to determine frequency, timings and triggers

Biological	Psychological
Pain, resulting from joint/dental/problems	Anxiety/fear
Discomfort due to skin, bowel problems, including constipation	Anger and/or frustration
Frontal lobe deficits leading to perseverative behaviours	Feels threatened
Response to hallucinations	Loneliness
Drug induced restlessness	Boredom
Infection induced confusion	Self-stimulate, particularly if deaf
Effects of alcohol	Over/under stimulated
Hunger/thirst	
Tiredness reducing threshold for irritability	

Social and environmental

Request for toilet

Request for food or drink

Requests are being ignored

Communication difficulties

Rejecting carers' approaches

Signalling dislike of someone in the vicinity

Attempt to annoy someone else

Excessive noise or silence

Recent change to environment

Immobile person sitting signalling discomfort – e.g. sitting in sunlight or in a draught

Rejection of current surroundings

Table 2.2 The common biopsychosocial causes of sexual disinhibition

Sexual disinhibition	
Biological	**Psychological**
Frontal lobe deficits, resulting in disinhibition	Bored
	Restless
Parkinson's medication resulting in hypersexuality	Misidentifying other people as one's partner
Excess use of alcohol, resulting in disinhibition	Believing one is young, and sexually available
High libido	Misinterpreting intimate personal care activities as a sexual advance
Social and environmental	Method of reducing stress
Lots of members of opposite sex in the environment	Disinhibition
Availability of bedrooms	A reliable method to be removed from a fearful/unwanted situation
Confused members of the opposite sex making advances	
Looking for companionship	
Looking for comfort	
Seeing other people in their night-wear	

Table 2.3 The common biopsychosocial causes of aggression

Aggression – one needs to observe such behaviours carefully as the label is very subjective. Many aggressive acts are the products of perceived threat and/or anxiety. Despite the destructive aspects, aggression indicates the person with dementia still feels things are worth fighting for. If she loses this self-belief, she may become depressed.

Biological	Psychological
Frontal lobe deficits	Restless
Head injury leading to disinhibition	Frustration at not being able to communicate well
Drug induced restlessness	Frustration at not being understood
Underlying physical conditions	Person thinks her rights are being infringed
Infection	Person feels patronised (treated like a child)
Effects of excess use of alcohol	Person thinks she is being unnecessarily rushed and harried
Paranoid delusions requiring someone to defend themselves	
Hallucinations requiring someone to defend themselves	Person thinks not being listened to
	Person feels embarrassed during personal care tasks
Pain reducing threshold of agitation	Person thinks her personal space is being invaded
Fending-off contact due to bodily pain	Person thinks not being allowed to use her existing abilities and skills
Temperament	Co-existent mental health problems
Sensory deficits	Disinhibition

Social and environmental

Culture

Misidentifying other people

Misperceiving other people's intentions

Interpersonal over-stimulation

A particular carer is not acceptable to her (e.g. due to age, gender, race or colour)

Person does not like being touched by someone else

Setting is unacceptable

Person not being allowed to leave the building

Person made to feel incompetent

Person does not like the restrictive rules and regulations being imposed

Caregivers providing inconsistent approaches

Over-stimulation (noise, lights)

Setting is too hot or cold

Weather is very warm and close

Table 2.4 The common biopsychosocial causes of stripping

Removing clothes (stripping) – environmental features (weather, room temperature), body temperature and cultural aspects play important roles with respect to this behaviour.

Biological	Psychological
Hypothalmus – temperature control impaired	Bored
	Restless
Frontal lobe deficits, resulting in disinhibition	Dislikes the clothes given to wear
	Protesting that clothes given are not their own clothes
Sensitive skin	
Drug-induced rash	Disinhibition
Drug-induced restlessness	Lifestyle preference (never worn many clothes)
Parkinson's medication resulting in hypersexuality	A method to be removed from a fearful situation
Underlying physical condition – resulting in feel hot	
High temperature due to infection	
Prostate problems	
Excess use of alcohol, feeling flushed and/or disinhibited	
Confusing night with day, thus undressing to prepare for bed	

Social and environmental

Copying other people

Preparing to engage in sexual acts

Culture does not wear many clothes, or does not regard nudity as a problematic issue

Setting is too hot

Weather is very warm and close

Person's room is very sunny

Preparation for going to the toilet

Clothes are irritable, itchy

Ill fitting clothes – too tight or loose

Underwear too tight

Chairs with surfaces that make people prone to sweating

Table 2.5 The common biopsychosocial causes of walking with/without purpose

Walking with/without purpose (wandering) – there are many positive aspects to this activity (exercise, stress reduction, etc.). Hence, it is often appropriate to provide safe walking areas, rather than deny people the opportunity to engage in the behaviour.

Biological	Psychological
Distraction from pain and discomfort	To reduce anxiety or fear
Relief physical discomfort (back pain, constipation)	Loneliness
Drug-induced restlessness	Boredom
Infection induced confusion	Over/under stimulated
Search for food or water due to hunger/thirst	Coping with distress
Sundowning	Exercise
Memory difficulties, resulting in people forgetting their original intentions	Enjoyment
Cognitive disorientation	To promote own sleep
	To give a sense of control
Social and environmental	Continuing a life-long habit
Searching for carer	Low mood
Searching for objects	To explore surroundings due to memory and orientation difficulties
Searching for family members	Walking after a meal
Searching for toilet	
Searching for own room	
Enables someone to meet others	
Poor signage	
Confused layout in setting	
Finding way to access garden	
Finding way out of building	
Orientate oneself to the surroundings	
Curious about environment	
Cues from light cycle (day/night)	

**Table 2.6 The common biopsychosocial
causes of absconding**

Absconding	
Biological	**Psychological**
Disorientation	Upset at having liberty taken away
Suspicious and paranoid about surroundings	Fear of staying in a strange place
Misperception that environment is hostile	Fear of being around confused people
	Looking for comfort and security
Social and environmental	Time displacement, thinking younger and person with care responsibilities
Environment is confusing	
Environment is dirty	
Environment is smelly, too hot	
Environment is under-stimulating	
Searching for family members	
Searching for object	
Searching for own room	
Enables someone to meet others	
Poor signage	
Confused layout in setting	
Unable to make friends in setting	
Finding way to access garden	
Finding way out of building	
Orientate oneself to the surroundings	
Curious about environment	
Cues from light cycle (day/night)	

Biopsychosocial causes of a range of BC

Tables such as Tables 2.1–2.6 above are helpful in providing ideas for treatment, and show the commonality of causes across the various types of BC. For example, pain may manifest itself behaviourally in numerous presentations from shouting to walking, and aggression. Thus to help clarify the specific causes of a BC, it is often beneficial to try to identify the idiosyncratic beliefs that may be driving the behaviour (e.g. I need to go home to collect the kids from school). This issue is discussed in more detail below.

ROLE OF BELIEFS

One of the chief ways NCBT's treatment differs from other methods in the field is its emphasis on the role of cognitions (thoughts and beliefs). Indeed, it is my opinion that beliefs play a key role in determining how disruptive a BC can become. It is relevant to note that even when clients' thinking becomes incoherent and muddled, one can often identify key beliefs that trigger and sustain their behaviours. Table 2.7 provides some examples of common motivating beliefs; note, they are described within the NCBT categorisation discussed in the first chapter in Table 1.2.

Table 2.7 Beliefs and thoughts associated with BCs

Type of BC	Beliefs and associated thoughts
Lack of motivation	Themes of hopelessness, negativity and learned helplessness: I am worthless; There's no point in trying, nothing changes; They never listen to what I want anyway.
Threat related	i. Themes of feeling vulnerable: I'm scared, I don't know where I am. This man thinks he's my husband. ii. Themes of perceived injustice and need to respond aggressively: They don't treat me with respect; You've got to stand-up for yourself. I'm not putting up with this!!
Information seeking	Themes of searching and making sense of things: Let me check this place out; If I go through there, maybe I'll find out where I am; I'll go and ask her where I am.

Table 2.7 Beliefs and thoughts associated with BCs *cont.*

Type of BC	Beliefs and associated thoughts
Failure to inhibit	Themes of impulsiveness and egocentric thinking: I want it straight away; She's got nice breasts; I want to be fed now.
Poor environmental fit	Themes of discomfort with current environment: I don't want to be here; This place stinks; The people here are old and weird.

By identifying these beliefs, and linking them with the background information, one is in a better position to understand the person's needs. In some situations the client's communication can be so poor that it is difficult to identify his thoughts. On such occasions, a clinician would work with the carer to hypothesise what the underlying beliefs might be. The method for generating hypotheses is discussed in Chapter 6.

To assist with collecting information about the causal factors a number of assessment tools can be used. Some of these scales and procedures are explained in the next section.

MEASURES

In the following discussion, I shall examine some of the tools that help identify the causal factors. Table 2.8 provides examples of the scales that can be used to assess the features discussed in the first section of this chapter. For an extensive review of scales used in the area, see Moniz-Cook *et al.* 2008a. All the tables referred to in Table 2.8 are presented at the end of this chapter.

Table 2.8 BC measures and tools

Feature	Types of measures and assessment tools
Cognition and neuropsychology	Common global assessments of functioning include the MMSE* and ADAS-cog. Global neuropsychological measures are also sometimes employed, such as the ACE-R, CDRS. Specific measures are common, particularly the executive assessments (e.g. BADS). Table 2.9 presents a scale developed in Newcastle to help staff assess clients' frontal lobe functioning. Scans are often useful, particularly the CT, DAT, and SPECT to identify areas of reduced functioning.
Drugs	It is helpful to keep a detailed record of people's present and past history of receiving medication. Older people tend to be prescribed a lot of medication in relation to mental and physical health issues. Consequently negative reactions to drugs might be missed, or blamed on other causes, because of failures to closely monitor people's drug histories.
Physical difficulties	Monitoring of vital signs (bloods, blood pressure, electrolytes, temperature, signs of infection) is common. Assessment of pain is particularly important, although difficult to assess in dementia (ADD; Cohen-Mansfield and Lipson 2002). A review by Stolee *et al.* (2005) favoured the use of DisDat and Pain Behaviour Measure. Other tools include: The Barthel ADL scale is useful for assessing people's functional and physical abilities. A screening tool currently under development by NCBT is presented in Table 2.10.
Perceptual deficits	In recent years researchers have found associations between deficits in smell, vision and auditory skills with cognitive decline (Gater *et al.* 2008). Problems of communication can sometimes lead clinicians to fail to identify visual and hearing problems. If suspected, help can be obtained from the relevant specialists.

Table 2.8 BC measures and tools cont.

Feature	Types of measures and assessment tools
Mental health	The Cornell Depression Scale and DMAS are good tools for assessing affective problems in people with dementia. The RAID is also a useful brief tool for assessing anxiety. The rAQ can be used to assess those people with long-standing social and communication difficulties, who've always required rigid routines in order to function.
Care practices	The DCM is helpful for examining staff interactions and features associated with clients' well-being. The QUIS is another useful observation tool, which examines carer's positive and negative interactions with clients.
Beliefs/emotions	Clients' beliefs and emotions are assessed using behavioural charts (see Figure 2.1). A more formal scale is currently under development by the NCBT to assess clients' beliefs and emotions (see Figure 2.2). From a carer's perspective, there are a number of scales that examine their beliefs and attitudes towards people with dementia (Formal Caregiver Attribution Inventory (Fopma-Loy 1991; Shirley 2005) and Controllability beliefs scale (Dagnan *et al.* 2004).

Table Key: ADAS-cog (Alzheimer's Disease Assessment Scale-cognitive sub-scale); ACER (Addenbrooke's Cognitive Examination Revised, Mioshi *et al.* 2006); ADD (Assessment of Discomfort in Dementia Scale, Kovach *et al.* 1999); rAQ (Relatives autism quotient, Baron-Cohen *et al.* 2001); BADS (Behavioural Assessment of the Dysexecutive Syndrome, Wilson *et al.* 1997); Barthel ADL (Mahoney and Barthel 1965); CDRS (Clinical Dementia Rating Scale, Hughes *et al.* 1982); Cornell depression scale (Alexopoulos *et al.* 1988); CT (Computerised tomography); DAT (Dopamine transporter scan); DCM (Dementia care mapping, Kitwood and Bredin 1992); DMAS (Dementia Mood Assessment Scale, Sunderland *et al.* 1998); DisDat (Discomfort in Dementia of Alzheimer's Type, Hurley *et al.* 2001); MMSE (Folstein *et al.* 1975); MRI (Magnetic resonance imaging); QUIS (Quality of interactions schedule, Dean *et al.* 1993); PBM (Pain Behaviour Measure, Keefe and Block 1982); RAID (Rating Anxiety in Dementia, Shankar *et al.* 1999); SPECT (Single positron emission computerised tomography).

In addition to these scales, there are a number of other useful assessment tools in relation to BC. One of the most relevant sets of scales identify the type and nature of the BC. Many assessment tools in this group are overly comprehensive and too lengthy to function well in a clinical setting. However, three that are suitable clinically are: Neuropsychiatric Inventory (NPI), Cohen-Mansfield Agitation Scale (CMAI, Cohen-Mansfield *et al.* 1989) and the Challenging Behaviour Scale (CBS, Moniz-Cook *et al.* 2001b).

The NPI has 12 sub-scales, 10 covering BC and two measuring neurovegatative conditions. Each sub-scale has an entry question about presence of symptoms. If this is answered positively, the full scale is completed; if the features are not present, the interviewer moves on to the next symptom cluster. The frequency and severity of symptoms over the month prior to interview are assessed and multiplied to produce a measure of severity. There are a number of versions, one of the most clinically useful contains a carer distress scale (Cummings *et al.* 1994; Kaufer *et al.* 1998). There are at least five versions of the CMAI (short form has 12 items, long 29 items). Four subtypes of agitation are identified: physical non-aggression; physical aggression; verbal non-aggression; verbal aggression. It is completed via face-face interviews with a carer.

The CBS is a 25-item scale designed to measure client behaviours (incidence, frequency, difficulty, and challenge) that carers find difficult to manage. It has been shown to have good validity and reliability and is completed by carers with assistance from clinicians. A helpful and comprehensive description of seven scales used to assess aggression in BC is provided by Johnson *et al.* (2008). Their article describes the features associated with scale selection.

For an overview of other relevant scales see Ballard *et al.* (2001); Burns *et al.* (1999) and Neville and Bryne (2001). It is important to note that many of the scales described in these reviews tend to be used in research rather than in day-to-day clinical work. With clinical relevance in mind, Figures 2.1 and 2.2 present two charts used by the NCBT to collect descriptive information from carers about the problematic behaviours. The first scale is a standard ABC behavioural chart, placing particular emphasis on recording clients' emotions.

Behavioural Chart for ....

Target behaviour .... Please record any episodes of the above behaviour (day/night). Aim – to record frequency and circumstances of incidents.	

Date and Time	What was the person doing just before the incident? **(A-antecedent)**
Where the incident occurred	
	What did you see happen? **(B- actual behaviour)**
Which staff were involved (initials)	

What did the person say at the time of the incident?

How did the person appear at the time of the incident? (maybe more than one tick)

Angry	☐		Frustrated	☐
Anxious	☐		Happy	☐
Bored	☐		Irritable	☐
Content	☐		Physically unwell	☐
Depressed	☐		Restless	☐
Despairing	☐		Sad	☐
Frightened	☐		Worried	☐

How was the situation resolved? **(C–consequences)** *

A – Antecedents are the features happening just prior to the emergence of the behaviour that may have served to trigger or reinforce it.

B – Behaviours are simply the factual acts witnessed by the staff. The staff are taught not to interpret the behaviour, rather provide factual details.

C – Consequences are the responses of others to the behavioural disturbance. An analysis of this aspect helps to determine what the person might be achieving by acting this way. Also by examining the consequences, one can check the behaviour is not being inadvertently reinforced. *Answers in this column give therapists ideas for interventions, and provide clues about which staff are dealing with the situation well (or not so well).

Figure 2.1 Example of a behavioural chart incorporating an ABC analysis together with elements of the Newcastle approach

Figure 2.2 describes a recent development that attempts to get staff to empathise with the beliefs of the client. The front page of the latter document has the following instructions:

Instructions for behavioural grid

Step 1: Identify the type of challenging behaviour (CB).

Step 2: Provide details about the CB incident; do this in two stages. First, give information about the CB, then include details about how other people *reacted* to it and any consequences.

Client's CB → Others' reactions to CB and consequences

Step 3: Use the 'Tables of Causes' [as in Tables 2.1–2.6] to identify reasons for the CBs.

Step 4: This step involves you imagining yourself in the position of the client. So try to guess what the client might've been thinking, and how these thoughts and beliefs led to the CB.

Step 5: Use your knowledge of both the client and the setting to *problem solve* the best way to deal with the CB.

Type of challenging behaviours	Description of challenging behaviours, including carers' reactions		Causes of the CB	Person's thoughts that triggered CB	Potential solutions
	CB	Reaction of others to the CB and the consequences			

Type of challenging behaviours	Description of challenging behaviours, including carers' reactions		Causes of the CB	Person's thoughts that triggered CB	Potential solutions
	CB	Reaction of others to the CB and the consequences			
Aggression	Peter put his hand on Mary's shoulder and asked her to sit next to him.	Nurse told Peter to leave Mary and pulled his hand from her shoulder. After this Peter hit the nurse in the mouth.	Owing to Peter misidentifying Mary as his wife due to his dementia, he is annoyed that she does not want to spend time with him. When the nurse takes his hand off Mary, Peter gets angry that someone else is interfering.	*This is my wife and she should be doing what I tell her to do.* And when nurse takes Peter's hand away… *Get off me, and keep out of my business with my wife.*	1. Currently Mary looks like his wife. So ask the hairdresser to colour her hair and change the style. 2. Bring in photographs of his wife, and continually orientate Peter to the picture. 3. Distract Peter e.g. ask him to help you unscrew top off a jar, and remove Mary from scene while he is doing this.

Figure 2.2 Challenging behaviour grid, incorporating carer reaction and beliefs (plus worked example)

Table 2.9 Frontal lobe functions

Difficulties	Practical description of difficulty
Perseveration	Repeating actions and statements over and over again.
Unable to inhibit responses	Unable to control aggressive or sexual actions/ statements that would normally be out of character.
Saying things to hurt other's feelings	Making unkind comments about others which can serve to provoke or upset them.
Impulsive actions and emotions	Suddenly doing something dangerous or risky – 'out of the blue'. Sudden outbursts of emotion.
Poor short-term/ working memory	Unable to correctly remember things done during the present day (e.g. breakfast, activities, etc.).
Recognition of objects, but unaware how to use them	Able to name an object, but unable to demonstrate its use (e.g. able to name a fork, but not aware how to use it).
Overly fixated on people or activities	Repeatedly paying attention, talking about or touching things (people, objects). Repetitive actions or activities.
Poor at making decisions	Unable to make choices, or decisions about what to do next (e.g. the person can't decide what he wants to wear or is unable to choose his food at meal times).
Poor planning	Unable to work out how to tackle a problem. For example, when a difficulty arises the client doesn't know where to begin, or can't grasp the nature of the problems (e.g. failing to move items off a table, before putting new ones on; doesn't recognise it would be helpful to write-out a shopping list prior to going shopping).

Poor sequencing	Unable to carry out actions in a logical sequence (e.g. unable to dress themselves in a logical order, or when toileting tends to open bowels prior to removing underwear).
Concrete thinking	Unable to think in an abstract way. Conversations tend to be interpreted in an overly direct manner (If told 'it will all come out in the wash', he/she thinks this refers to washing clothes).
Confabulation	Prone to giving stories and/or explanations in order to fill in gaps in his/her memory.
Lack of insight	Unaware of his current difficulties and limitations. Not being aware of the risks associated with these limitations (e.g. failing to appreciate he would not be able to live by himself at home).
Poor concentration	Unable to concentrate on anything for an extended period of time (e.g. watching TV, reading). Client's focus tends to move quickly on to something else.
Distractibility	Easily distracted by things going on in the environment. When undertaking a task will lose interest in the task if interrupted by someone or something (e.g. a sound).
Apathy	Emotionally unresponsive, even when being provoked.
Euphoria	Overly enthusiastic, and/or inappropriately laughing out loud.

Table Key: Item is rated on 1–5 scale (not like person–totally like person).

Table 2.10 Some of the potential causal factors that are screened at referral

Key area	Type of problem	Example of problem which may be causal factor in BC
Age related issues	Sensory difficulties	Sight, hearing difficulties
	Pain	Arthritis, dental pain
Physiological and physical problems	Delerium	Confusion
	Constipation	Discomfort, problematic gait, irritability
	Seizures	Confusion
	Vascular events	Sudden deterioration in skills
	Infections	UTI, cellulitis
	Diabetes	Variable levels of insight/performance
	Cancer	Brain metastases
	Thyroid	Hyper (agitated), hypo (confused)
Mental health problems	Psychosis	Hallucinations, delusions
	Depression	Irritability, labile, sleep problems
	Anxiety	Reassurance seeking
	Other	OCD, social phobia, trauma

Medication	Anti-psychotics	Confusion
	Benzodiazepines	Over-sedation
	Parkinson's meds	Hypersexuality
	Pain relief	Constipation
	Statins	Agitation
Environment	Confusion, disorientation, boredom	Noise, bright light, smell, crowding
Premorbid personality	Temperament and development	Learning disability, autism, difficult personality trait

Table 2.11 Cognitive deficits that may be causal factors in BC

Key cognitive area	Type of skill difficulty
Memory	Inability to lay down new memories (STM deficits) leading to forgetting what just been told or done.
	Recognition difficulties, misidentifying objects or people.
Frontal difficulties	Impulsiveness, disinhibition, apathy.
	Sequencing, planning, impaired, judgement and decision making (see Table 2.9).
Poor orientation	Inability to indicate the date, their age and/or name where they are.
Poor level of insight	Unaware of the extent of their difficulties, or abilities to look after self, thus may engage in risky behaviours.
Poor attention and concentration	Unable to focus, easily distracted.
Deficits in emotional regulation	Excessive laughing or weepiness.
Difficulties in communicating needs	Receptive and expressive problems, leading to frustration and agitation.

Note: A full assessment involves examining the person's history and life-preferences, and undertaking a detailed analysis of the behavioural difficulties. More detailed assessments of some of the features outlined in the table may also need to be undertaken.

Chapter 3

Using Psychotropic Medication to Treat Challenging Behaviour

INTRODUCTION

Risperidone, an atypical anti-psychotic, is the only psychotropic medication licensed to treat challenging behaviour. Even then, its use should be restricted to those people with moderate to severe Alzheimer's disease who are displaying persistent aggression that may result in harm to themselves or others. The licence is for short-term use (6 weeks) and assumes non-pharmacological treatments have been tried previously. Therefore, when a medical practitioner is using any drug other than risperidone, she is prescribing 'off-licence', and thus the medication must be used with caution. However, neither caution nor restraint characterise the history of prescribing in this area (Ballard *et al.* 2009). For example, according to Holland (2008) there is a long history of excessive and inappropriate use of major tranquillising medication (anti-psychotics) for BC, the logic being that someone being aggressive and/or shouting requires 'tranquillising'. The view that tranquillisation and sedation have been over-used is echoed in many major reviews (Ballard *et al.* 2009; Sink *et al.* 2005; Schneider *et al.* 2005), national guidelines (National Dementia Strategy for England, DoH 2009) and UK government reports (All-Party Parliamentary Group on Dementia 2008; Banerjee 2009). However, despite such misgivings, it is important to recognise that medication plays an extremely important role in the treatment of BC, particularly when used to treat the underlying causes of the behaviour (pain, seizures, infections, depression, psychosis), and when used in accordance with the protocol outlined in Chapter 1, Figure 1.2.

By the end of this chapter the reader will be aware of the following:

- The types of psychotropic medications given to treat BC, and an overview of their side-effects.

- There is a poor evidence-base underpinning the use of the classes of drugs.

- There are a number of guidelines influencing prescribing practices.

- Alternative approaches to medication are available, but advice about their use is generally poor.

GENERAL ISSUES

The use of psychotropics in the treatment of BC has received a great deal of attention of late due to increasing evidence calling into question their effectiveness, and major worries about their side-effects. Indeed, there are now questions about whether such medications, particularly the anti-psychotics, are being used in client's best interests (Mental Capacity Act, 2005). These concerns are leading to fears of litigation and worries about complaints from families and advocates.

Prescribing in this area has always been difficult, which is in part due to the slower metabolising abilities of older people, leading to a higher degrees of toxicity at lower doses. However, most of the problematic side-effects are due to the powerful generic impact of some of these drugs on people's bodies. Polypharmacy is also a concern, with many older people taking numerous different medications for various physical and mental health conditions. There is also increasing concerns about polypharmacy within the same class of drugs. For example, a recent edition of 'The Psychiatrist' (Taylor 2010) was dedicated to the largely disapproved of practice of multi-prescribing of anti-psychotics. In relation to prescribing for people with dementia, the situation is rather complex because some conditions are under-diagnosed and under-treated (e.g. pain, depression), while others are over-medicated (e.g. BC). If the above issues did not complicate matters enough, the situation is made worse by frequent reports of mis-prescribing and maladministration of the drugs, particularly in care settings (Barber 2009). Barber's survey found that 70 per cent of residents in care had experienced at least one drug error, usually in the form of an administration, or dispensing, or a prescribing error. The errors were attributed to the following reasons: doctors being inaccessible or not knowing the residents, high workloads of staff, lack of training of staff and pharmacists, and poor teamwork and record keeping. There is also a particular emphasis on improving the prescribing practices of primary care doctors (e.g. general practitioners, GPs), who do not have the same support, expertise and resources that are available to their colleagues in secondary care. Indeed, owing to the complexity involved in prescribing for BC, concerns about deaths and fears of litigation, some GPs are no longer willing to prescribe for challenging presentations.

PSYCHOTROPIC DRUGS USED IN THE TREATMENT OF CHALLENGING BEHAVIOURS

An overview and brief description of the main medications used to treat BC is presented, followed by some comments about each class of drug (see Table 3.1).

Anti-psychotics

It is estimated that 30–40 per cent of residents with dementia develop psychosis with paranoid delusions or hallucinations at some time during the course of their illness; these experiences may be short-lived and can resolve spontaneously. In most situations where the symptoms persist, the appropriate treatment is a short spell on an anti-psychotic. Unfortunately, these powerful tranquillisers tend to be given when there is no evidence of a psychosis, and once prescribed the drugs are often not withdrawn. For example, prior to the introduction of guidelines in 1987 in the USA, it was estimated that 43–55 per cent of residents in care were receiving anti-psychotics. In UK surveys of *nursing* homes, it was found that between 24 per cent (McGrath and Jackson 1996) and 36 per cent (Dempsey and Moore 2005) of residents were prescribed such medication. In *residential* homes, the rate of prescribing was also high, at 29 per cent (Dempsey and Moore 2005).

Table 3.1 List of medications used to treat challenging behaviours

Medication	Intended purpose
Anti-psychotic (aka neuroleptic, major tranquilliser drugs): *Typical* (e.g. haloperidol, chlorpromazine, promazine) *Atypical* (e.g. quetiapine, amisulphride, risperidone, olanzapine)	These are powerful drugs used to treat psychosis, but are believed to be useful in controlling aggression, agitation resulting from unwanted hallucinations and delusions in dementia. Two types – 'typicals', which are the older class of drugs. They tend to have more side-effects than the 'atypicals'. The newer types tend to be less sedative. Anti-psychotics should not be used for certain types of dementia, such as dementia with Lewy body, due to the potential for severe side-effects.
Benzodiazepines/ sedatives (e.g. lorazepam, diazepam, nitrazapam, temazepam)	Drugs used to sedate and promote sleep. Often used when there is no evidence of psychotic features. They are effective over short time scales only, and there are problems with dependency and falls.
Anti-depressants (e.g. citalopram, trazodone, sertraline, mirtazapine)	Drugs used to treat apathy and depression as a discrete disorder. They are also used to treat BC, owing to the sedative effects of some of the anti-depressants.
Anti-convulsants (carbamazepine, sodium valproate, gabapentin)	These anti-epileptic drugs reduce excessive electrical activity in the brain to restore normal functioning.
Anti-dementia drugs, such as the acetyl-cholinesterase inhibitors (donepezil, rivastigmine, galantamine) and memantine	Drugs originally used to slow down cognitive decline and enhance cognitive performance of people diagnosed with dementia. Preliminary evidence suggests they may be effective in treating some behavioural problems. The cholinesterase inhibitors seem to help with apathy and memantine with agitation.

These rates are particularly worrying owing to the modest level of evidence for the efficacy of this medication in the treatment of BC. In a systematic review, which examined five well-controlled trials assessing atypical anti-psychotics, limited evidence was obtained in favour of their use (Lee *et al.* 2004). A more recent review (Ballard *et al.* 2009), examining the evidence for agitation and aggression only, noted that while there were no benefits in terms of long-term use of the drugs (6 months plus), there was some evidence of short-term efficacy in relation to aggression. Banerjee (2009) calculated that only 20 per cent of people (36,000 cases per year) benefit from the use of anti-psychotics. Further, the authors of the various reviews have cautioned against the use of anti-psychotics due to their well-documented side-effects, such as an increased mortality rate, risk of falls, drowsiness, Parkinsonism, movement disorders, drug sensitivity reactions and accelerated intellectual decline (McShane *et al.* 1997). Furthermore, there are specific concerns about the cardiotoxicity of thioridazine, and the increased risk of cerebrovascular events in patients taking risperidone and olanzapine (Schneider *et al.* 2005). The risk profile for anti-psychotics is presented in Figure 3.1. Such risks can be minimised by keeping to the lowest dose and careful monitoring of how much medication is needed.

A list of clinical recommendations regarding how these drugs should be used is provided by Ballard *et al.* (2009); one of the principles being: 'Use of these drugs should probably be restricted to short-term management (up to 12 weeks) of severe physical aggression' (p.249). The most recent national guidance on the topic has come from a UK government commissioned review written for the UK Minister of State for Care Services ('Time for Action', Banerjee 2009). Banerjee has called for a reduction in the prescribing of anti-psychotics, setting the ambitious target of a reduction of up to 66 per cent over a 36-month period, starting in January 2010. The DoH document contains 11 recommendations, including a call for strong national and local leadership, use of medication audits, better inspection processes, staff training, use of preventative strategies, etc.

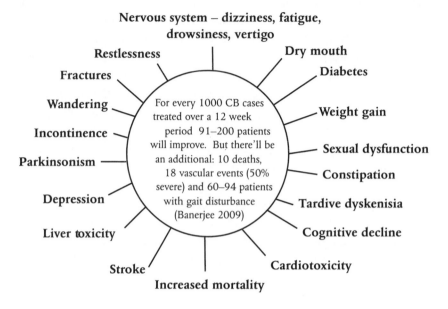

Figure 3.1 Anti-psychotic side-effects

Benzodiazepines (sedatives)

Benzodiazepines are used to treat BC, either alone or in combination with anti-psychotics. As benzodiazepines are sedatives, they are commonly used to reduce anxiety, agitation and promote sleep. There is growing evidence that their use has increased in recent years due to the criticisms levelled at anti-psychotics (Bishara *et al.* 2009). Bishara's survey of UK Trusts' prescribing patterns provided evidence that, although not viewed as the most effective class of drug for BC, on some wards they are the most commonly used.

Despite some favourable findings (Meehan *et al.* 2002), case reports and anecdotal evidence suggest that benzodiazepines can lead to increased agitation, confusion and falls in dementia (Hogan, Maxwell, Fung and Ebly 2003; Wagner *et al.* 2004). On balance, Sink *et al.* (2005) suggest that benzodiazepines should be avoided in the treatment of BC, especially for long-term management. The latter view is an echo of an earlier report published by the Expert Consensus Panel for Agitation in Dementia (1998), which recommended that benzodiazepines should not be prescribed except for occasional, short-term use to relieve anxiety.

Anti-depressants

Anti-depressants are often used to treat both apathy and depression in people with dementia, and it could be argued that they are under-used for these purposes. In people with dementia, depression can be associated with increasing irritability and worsening concentration and therefore may be a cause or exacerbating factor of a BC. Some of the new anti-depressants are helpful in treating sleep and appetite disorders, anxiety and obsessive behaviours. When choosing which anti-depressant to use, consideration needs to be given to the exact characteristics of the person's presentation and the potential impact – including side-effects, such as stomach upset, dry mouth, constipation, blurred vision and dizziness, weight gain, and associated diabetes.

Pollock *et al.* (2002) report that some psychotic symptoms respond to the use of anti-depressants. Clearly this effect may be indirect because many people experiencing psychosis display comorbid depressive features (Steinberg and Lyketsos 2005). Pollock *et al.*'s (2002) study was one of the few RCTs to have shown an anti-depressant (citalopram) to be beneficial in the treatment of BC. This trial resulted in a significant reduction on the Neurobehavioural Rating Scale (NRS) for hospitalised patients in terms of agitation and lability (Levin *et al.* 1987). In summary, based on the findings of Sink *et al.*'s systematic review, which identified five quality studies, the available evidence is that anti-depressants are largely ineffective for BC when depression is not present; although a recent review by Ballard *et al.* (2009) again makes the case for using citalopram for the treatment of agitation.

Anti-convulsants

Whilst a less common treatment for BC, these drugs are used when there are signs of episodic outbursts and epileptic seizures. In other situations they appear to offer few benefits (Sink *et al.* 2005), but may also cause problematic effects (e.g. drowsiness) (Tariot *et al.* 2001; Sival *et al.* 2002). Porteinsson *et al.* (2001) reported no differences between sodium valproate and placebo groups, but adverse effects such as sedation, weakness and respiratory problems in the drug group. In Sink's review, she found that the three RCT trials that had investigated the use of valproate revealed a lack of efficacy with its use (Sink *et al.* 2005). A more up-to-date review of the anti-convulsants supports this view (Ballard *et al.* 2009), although it notes that there is preliminary evidence emerging for the use of carbamazepine in the treatment of agitation and aggression. It is relevant to note that the use of these drugs has its problems, because they are toxic and can interact negatively with other drugs commonly used with elderly patients.

Anti-dementia drugs

Ballard et al.'s (2009) review suggests that the cholinesterase inhibitors may be helpful in the treatment of agitation and apathy, above and beyond their normal role as cognitive enhancers. In support of this case he cites a meta-analytic review (Trinh, Hoblyn, Mohanty and Yaffe 2003) and a withdrawal study which found that withdrawing donepezil resulted in a significant worsening in behavioural problems (Holmes et al. 2004). However, the jury remains out with respect to this class of drugs as a large RCT study failed to find any BC benefits over a 12-week period (see Ballard et al. 2009).

Encouraging results are beginning to emerge with the use of memantine, although no well-controlled RCT trials have been conducted. According to Ballard et al. (2009), memantine may prove to be an effective alternative to the use of anti-psychotics for some individuals presenting with agitation. However, such optimism may be a little premature because much of the current evidence in support of the drug comes from pooled data from different studies (Gauthier, Wirth and Mobius 2005; McShane, Areosa Sastre and Minakaran 2006).

It is noteworthy that the present review has focused on psychotropic medications, but other drugs are useful in maintaining clients' well-being. For example, Cohen-Mansfield (2006) has shown that the pain relief can lead to significant reductions in BC. In her study, many of the clients were not complaining of pain, but were prescribed medication following a review of their physical status by a medical practitioner. The rationale for prescribing was based on the doctor's considered opinion that the person was likely to be experiencing pain, due to arthritis, chronic back pain, fractures, etc.

DISCUSSION

Currently there are numerous concerns amongst medical clinicians about how to treat BC, with requests for both clearer guidance from professional bodies and help to standardise practice (Bishara et al. 2009).

This call was highlighted in a survey entitled the 'Expert Opinion Survey' that targeted all Consultant Old Age Psychiatrists in the UK (Bishara *et al.* 2009); response rate 35 per cent (n = 59). Its aim was to investigate current prescribing practices, by providing three vignettes for which the participants needed to state the appropriateness of a range of medication. In the first vignette the patient had psychosis associated with dementia, the second described signs of aggression and agitation, and in the third case there was a mixed presentation of screaming, wandering and disinhibition. The results are summarised in Table 3.2 in terms of the top five drugs deemed appropriate in each of the three vignettes.

Table 3.2 The top five psychotropics chosen for Bishara's three vignettes

Psychosis	Agitation and aggression	Screaming, wandering, disinhibition
Quetiapine	Quetiapine	Quetiapine
Acetylcholinesterases	Benzodiazepines	Trazadone
Amisulphride	Amisulphride	Benzodiazapines
Benzodiazepines	Trazadone	Acetylcholinesterases
Risperidone	Acetylcholinesterases	Amisulphride

In addition to getting the psychiatrist to rate what they thought was appropriate, a further arm of Bishara's study asked pharmacists from selected sites to provide a snap-shot view of prescribing for BC on hospital wards. The pharmacy results were somewhat inconsistent to the psychiatrists' self-reporting because the benzodiazepines were the class of medication most frequently requested.

Such inconsistencies are well recognised in this area (Jackson 2005). Therefore, a number of good practice BC guidelines have been published (e.g. Omnibus Reconciliation Act OBRA 87, Slater and Glazer 1995; Lantz *et al.* 1996; SIGN 1998; Howard *et al.* 2001; DoH 2009b). The OBRA guidelines were enacted in the USA, restricting the use of anti-psychotics in people with dementia. These guidelines also recommend that the responsibility of monitoring medication should be with the care facility rather than the prescribing physician. Since OBRA was introduced, the use of anti-psychotic medication has reduced by a third in the US. UK guidelines (Howard *et al.* 2001) recommend that unless a problem is causing severe distress or puts the person or others at risk, psychological or environmental management options should be the first line approach. Furthermore, as many challenging symptoms are transient and recover spontaneously, it is recommended that a discontinuation of pharmacological treatments occur after symptoms have been absent, or are minimal, for 3 months. As noted earlier, the latest UK government recommendations call for a 66 per cent reduction in the use of anti-psychotics, and the progress towards this goal will be monitored on a yearly basis (Banerjee 2009). To achieve such a goal, Banerjee's DoH report calls for local clinicians to show leadership in improving the situation for people displaying BCs. A good example of a recent initiative in relation to guidelines is the development of the Hampshire Partnership Foundation Trust Prescribing Guidelines (Holmes 2009). In this open access document, Holmes provides treatment guidance in relation to specific types of BC, making use of the evidence of McShane *et al.* (1997) and Gauthier *et al.* (2008) that certain behaviours form clusters and these groupings respond differently to the various classes of medication (e.g. the apathy cluster responds better to cholinesterase inhibitors). Figure 1.2 in Chapter 1 is based on Holmes' protocol, sharing many of the recommendations, although giving more serious consideration to the use of non-pharmacological approaches. Indeed, the Holmes paper, while providing detailed descriptions of medications and dosages, gives cursory guidance in terms of psychological approaches. This is an unfortunate omission as much greater specification is required in this matter, because if treatment protocols are serious about using psychological methods, they need to provide direction and leadership.

Finally, evidence shows us that psychiatrists are acutely aware of the problems associated with psychotropics. They think that have been put in a difficult position by current guidelines (Bishara *et al.* 2009), particularly with the need to reduce their use of anti-psychotics by two-thirds. Many of them feel that the national guidelines are unrealistic and unworkable unless there is significant investment in the field (Wood-Mitchell *et al.* 2008; Bishara *et al.* 2009). To highlight the current situation, here is a quote from the Expert Opinion Survey:

From our survey, it appears that the use of pharmacological agents for the management of BPSD does not appear to be favoured by the experts [the psychiatrists]. They remarked that they would rather have effective and adequate nursing input and use non-pharmacological options where possible but the scarce availability of these options is a major limiting factor for their use... There seems to be a national need for more resources so as to invest in adequate staff numbers, effective training and appropriate facilities for managing patients with BPSD, without resorting to medication. (Bishara *et al.* 2009, pp.951–2)

This quote is a positive statement in support of non-pharmacological approaches. However, what is needed in the field is not a monopoly by any one mode of treatment over another, rather a combined approach which makes best use of the various methodologies. To achieve this, clinicians need to think through the mechanisms by which change is likely to be achieved, and then deliver the treatments accordingly. For example, take the case of Mr Jones who is both depressed and aggressive. After formulating his difficulties, our 'change mechanism' for him is to first treat his depression prior to using some behavioural strategies for his aggression. This is because his depression is currently too severe to permit him to engage in any form of meaningful relationship with either therapists or carers.

CONCLUSION

Despite Banerjee's (2009) helpful recommendations on the use of anti-psychotics, I do not think it is too alarmist to suggest that the whole area of prescribing for BC is in a state of crisis. There are inconsistencies between protocols, concerns about efficacy and side-effects, and worries about potential litigation from confused and angry families. The situation is also not helped by the lack of specificity regarding the alternatives to medication. Indeed, currently non-pharmacological treatments are suggested as a first-line treatment, but this proposal is somewhat unrealistic until better guidance is provided.

Until directives on psychological treatments are improved, we are left chiefly with medication options. However, due to their ineffectiveness, it could be argued that it's unethical to use psychotropics unless used in conjunction with a non-pharmacological approach. Pharmacological guidelines and algorithms inform us that in those situations where pharmacotherapy is considered necessary, it should be tailored to the individual (Gill 2005). And according to Jackson (2005), all the drugs should be carefully monitored and reviewed in order to detect side-effects, and assessed regularly concerning whether the person still requires the medication and dose in question. Jackson summarises his approach to the use of medication as: start low; go slow; regular reviews; stop as soon as possible.

Chapter 4

Psychological and Other Non-pharmacological Approaches

INTRODUCTION

The role of non-pharmacological models in the treatment of BC has been highlighted in international (Vernooij-Dassen *et al.* 2010) and national reports and guidelines (National Dementia Strategies 2009, 2010; NICE Guidelines for Dementia 2006; National Service Framework for Older People, DoH 2001; Everybody's Business, DoH 2005). Such calls are also consistent with the recent push for giving all people, whatever their status or disability, better access to psychological therapies (DoH 2009b). However, despite there being a clear need for the use of non-pharmacological treatments, there is little agreement about which ones to use. Further, notwithstanding a long history of using psychological treatments in this area, their evidence-base in relation to BC remains poor. Orrell and Woods (1996) suggest that this lack of evidence makes it difficult for commissioners to plan services, and prevents comparisons being made with pharmacological regimens. This chapter provides readers with a review of the area, and suggests that slowly the evidence is increasing in relation to the use of psychological treatments (Livingston *et al.* 2005).

By the end of this chapter the reader will be aware of the following:

- BC are mostly managed well by staff as part of their routine care. As such, the majority of the non-pharmacological interventions are carried out by experienced carers without assistance from specialist teams.

- There are many psychological approaches, but few have a good evidence-base.

- It is important to distinguish between preventative approaches and interventions. Interventions are used to treat BC once they have emerged.

- Quality interventions tend to be formulation-led strategies tailored to the specific needs of the person within the setting. They often take the form of relatively simple actions (e.g. placing a sign on a door; allowing someone to eat by himself rather than in a large communal room; providing access to a garden).

- Success in using psychological approaches is highly dependent on how well they are delivered, and therefore it is important to support carers in delivering the interventions.

NON-PHARMACOLOGICAL APPROACHES IN GENERAL

Figure 4.1 outlines the positioning of non-pharmacological approaches in the treatment of people with BC. As stated previously, BC are common occurrences, and carers quickly become accustomed to dealing with them. Hence, in terms of frequency, carer management strategies are the most frequently used of the non-pharmacological approaches. Examples of these include: distraction and diversion (asking someone who is requesting to go out, to help you wash some dishes); de-escalation (encouraging someone who is angry to walk in the garden); opportunism (waiting until someone is passing the toilet before suggesting she may want to go); provision of alternative goals (giving a person who likes to dismantle furniture, blocks of wood and sand-paper); deception (purposefully hiding items that are known to make someone distressed or aggressive). Over time carers can become very skilled in using such management strategies. [NB. part of the work of specialist clinicians is often to identify good practices, work-out why they are beneficial, and then get carers to adopt the methods in a more systematic and routine manner. This is the methodology used by NCBT, and it will be explained in detail in Chapter 5.] In relation to Figure 4.1, there are four other non-pharmacological options (items 2–4). This chapter mainly addresses the psychological strategies (item 3). However, it is important to briefly acknowledge the role of the other two features (items 2 and 4), which are also discussed elsewhere in this book.

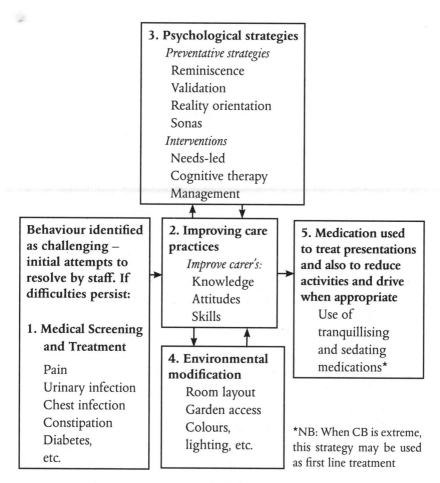

Figure 4.1 The position of the non-pharmacological approaches in the treatment of BC

IMPROVING CARE PRACTICES

The main theme of this book relates to enhancing care practices, and this is because carers play such an important role in the lives of people with moderate to severe dementia. Carers are involved in many personal care activities, assisting with dressing and toileting, shaving, feeding, etc. Such close contact, around potentially embarrassing issues, is often a source of frustration and a frequent trigger for BC. Hence, training carers to interact and communicate better when helping clients engage in activities of daily living is considered important (Levy-Storms 2008). When attempting to enhance care practices (i.e. refining existing strategies and/or developing new ones) therapists often refer to a three-pronged attack: facilitating changes in knowledge, attitudes and skills. As such, many training programmes target these three features, as illustrated in the work done in teaching carers better communication techniques (Finnema *et al.* 2005; van Weert *et al.* 2005, 2006). In these various programmes, carers are taught about the nature of dementia, use of non-verbal skills, facilitation of resident-to-resident communication, 'approach' strategies, disengagement strategies, etc. A systematic review of the use of communication strategies in dementia care settings showed positive results (Vasse *et al.* 2010), indicating that carers can improve their communication styles; although, these improvements were not always associated with reductions in the incidence of BC (McGilton *et al.* 2009). Figure 4.2 presents some key features to help improve care communication. For a comprehensive list of communication features see Dynes (2009).

When I first started working in the field of dementia, having read the literature on teaching, I organised a number of training courses for care staff in homes. However, it soon became apparent that the issues were far more complicated than the articles would lead one to believe. Indeed, sometimes the training was counterproductive because the experienced staff in the care homes felt patronised by the contents of the training. Such staff often had an extremely good knowledge-base, although they usually did not have the awareness of the specific terminology of the concepts they were using. And, in relation to skills, if one asked them what they would do in a challenging scenario, they would frequently generate sensible therapeutic suggestions. Furthermore, in many cases, there would be a resident within the care setting to whom the staff would currently be giving skilled person-centred care (NB. such residents would often be referred to as 'their favourite residents'). Hence, it was evident that the staff as a group had good knowledge and skills. Based on such insight, it occurred to me that the challenge in using non-pharmacological approaches was often *not* teaching carers 'What to do?' rather it was training them 'How to implement their approaches successfully for *all* residents and not just for their favourites'. Moreover, recognising that staff often knew what to do in many BC situations caused me to become interested in the reasons why their knowledge and skills were not better utilised. Following reflection, and from work undertaken with the Alzheimer's Society (Fossey and James 2007), I began to understand some of the 'obstacles to change'; some of which included: poor leadership, task-focused work-targets, inadequate staffing ratios, poor communication, including the effects of staff with a poor

METHOD OF COMMUNICATING

Speak slowly and distinctly in a quiet place, using short sentences. Use non-verbal gestures to assist understanding. Approach the person from the front, use good eye-contact and get down to her level if she's seated. Identify yourself and use client's name and summarise frequently.

CONTENTS OF COMMUNICATION

Avoid asking too many questions. Avoid questions that rely too heavily on memory or problem solving. Simple questions requiring Yes/No replies can be helpful. Keep things positive. Speak about emotions rather than arguing over facts. Avoid correcting the client when possible. Many of the above skills are outlined in the Qualification and Credit Framework for dementia: www.qcda.gov.uk

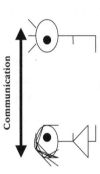

Communication

CLIENT

Use hearing and visual aids. If needed, ensure client's teeth fit well to aid speech. Ensure she is free from pain, discomfort and her basic physical needs are met e.g. there are no infections, nor conditions that will interfere with her concentration and ability to engage with others. Ensure client is not over-medicated, and not suffering side-effects.

CARER

Carers need the time and skills to work well with the client, including knowledge of psychological strategies. They must demonstrate respect, promote autonomy, be able to engage client in pleasant stimulating activities. Know how to break down complex tasks into simple components. Have the patience to employ simple and predictable routines. Ability to reassure the client, also be able to distract, redirect, comfort and use these various methods flexibly.

ENVIRONMENT

Appropriate lighting, acoustics, signage, opportunities for activities. Use of stimulating, safe and secure environmental design. Access to open and outside areas. Provision of areas where clients can go to avoid over-stimulation. Provide good access to family and friends, and provide area for family to visit.

The chairs, beds, table, etc. need to be comfortable, and the rooms personalised. Areas should not be over-crowded. Use of simple user-friendly designs of door knobs, sinks, handles to promote independence.

There should be sufficient carer/staff ratios and resources to promote psychological well-being in addition to good physical care.

ORGANISATIONS

Positive philosophy and attitude towards clients and others who are involved in the caring process. Opportunities for training and advancement of carers. Good relationship with NHS, Social services and inspectors. Access to funding for equipment and training. Good communication with, and access to, appropriate professionals.

When client is still in *own home*, carer needs to be advised and supported, and may require respite during course of the client's illness, or When client is in a *care facility*, her well-being is improved when home has good leadership and management structures. In such facilities there also needs to be investment in staff in order to prevent high turn-over.

Figure 4.2 Promoting good 2-way interactions: the wedding cake model

command of English, etc. It is evident that such issues can lead to staff stress, poor morale, high staff turnover, depersonalisation of the residents, and a loss of interest in the needs of the people staff are caring for. Thus as the various forms of psychological strategies are described below, it is important to keep these obstacles in mind and to empathise with the difficulties in implementing the non-pharmacological approaches.

ENVIRONMENTAL MODIFICATION

A comprehensive evidence-base has yet to be established in this area (Hulme *et al.* 2010; Zuidema *et al.* 2010), although a number of controlled studies (see Livingston *et al.* 2005) and a larger number of non-controlled studies have shown environment and design to be important (Judd, Marshall and Phippen 1997). The use of appropriate colour schemes and signposting in an environment can help with orientation and discrimination (Gibson *et al.* 2004). Designing an environment with a more home-like atmosphere with good lighting and some environmental stimulation can reduce agitation (Day *et al.* 2000). Access to safe gardens and outdoor spaces is also beneficial and opens up the possibility to develop horticultural type therapies with residents. BC occur less often in nursing homes with visual designs near exit doors (e.g. striped lines), and where there is more privacy (Zeisel *et al.* 2003). A sensory-enriched psychosocial environment is associated with low levels of agitation (Sloane *et al.* 1998).

PSYCHOLOGICAL METHODS

In Cohen-Mansfield's (2001) systematic review of psychological treatments, she classified eight types of intervention: sensory, social contact (real or simulated), behaviour therapy, staff training, structured activities, environmental interventions, medical/nursing care interventions and combination therapies. She identified 83 non-pharmacological intervention studies via her search, although many were of a poor standard. Table 4.1 provides an overview of some of the traditional psychological approaches used with older people. These methods have been reviewed systematically using the rigorous Cochrane research criteria. The Cochrane reports are systematic reviews concerning the evidence supporting specific treatments. They are particularly important to providers of services because commissioners in the UK frequently use them as a guide to what is suitable to fund. Cochrane reviews are also important in helping inform national recommendations and guidelines.

Table 4.1 Non-pharmacological approaches and their evidence-base

I Generic therapies	Systematic reviews and empirical status	Key articles
Reality orientation: uses rehearsal and physical prompts to improve cognitive functioning related to personal orientation.	A Cochrane review by Spector *et al.* (2002) identified six RCTs. The reviewers concluded there was evidence of improvements in terms of cognitive and behavioural features. RO is now assessed under Cognitive Stimulation Therapy.	Holden and Woods (1982); Holt *et al.* 2003; Verkaik *et al.* (2005)
Reminiscence therapy: involves discussion of past experiences individually or in a group format. Photographs, familiar objects, or sensory items used to prompt recall.	A Cochrane review by Woods *et al.* (2005b, updated 2009) identified five RCTs, four containing extractable data. The reviewers reported significant results in terms of cognitions, mood, caregiver strain and functional abilities. However, the quality of the studies was perceived to be poor.	Gibson (1994); Bohlmeijer *et al.* (2003)
Validation therapy: based on the general principle of acceptance of the reality of the person and validation of his/her experience.	A Cochrane review by Neal and Barton Wright (2003, updated 2009) identified three studies, two showing positive effects. However, the reviewers concluded there was insufficient evidence to view the approach as effective.	Finnema *et al.* (2005), Schrijnemaekers *et al.* (2002)
Psychomotor therapy: exercises (e.g. walking and ball games) are used to target depression and behavioural difficulties.	A Cochrane review by Montgomery and Dennis (2002) examining the impact of exercise on sleep problems identified one trial that demonstrated significant effects on a range of sleep variables. Forbes *et al.* 2008 found limited evidence that physical exercise slowed down cognitive decline.	Winstead-Fry and Kijek (1999); Hopman-Rock *et al.* (1999)

Table 4.1 Non-pharmacological approaches and their evidence-base cont.

I Generic therapies	Systematic reviews and empirical status	Key articles
Multi-sensory stimulation: stimuli such as light, sound and tactile sensations, often in specially designed rooms, used to increase the opportunity for communication and improved quality of experience.	A Cochrane review by Chung and Lai (2002, updated 2009) identified two RCTs. Despite some favourable results, the studies were so different that they could not be pooled. As such, the reviewers concluded there was insufficient evidence to view the approach as effective.	Baker *et al.* (2001); Van Weert *et al.* (2005)
Cognitive stimulation therapy: derived from reality orientation, focuses on information processing rather than rehearsal of factual knowledge.	Awaiting findings of a new review by Woods *et al.* (2009). The two previous reviews (Clare *et al.* 2003; Woods *et al.* 2005a) concluded that despite positive evidence there was insufficient evidence to view the approach as effective.	Clare *et al.* 2003; Woods *et al.* 2005a; Spector *et al.* (2003, 2006)
Aromatherapy: use of essential oils to provide sensory experiences and interactions with staff. The oils can be administered via massage techniques or in patients' baths.	A Cochrane review by Holt *et al.* (2003) identified two RCTs, but only Ballard *et al.* (2002) trial reviewed. This trial, despite flaws, was viewed favourably in terms of reducing agitation and neuropsychiatric symptoms. Quynh-anh and Patons' (2008) work showed equivocal results.	Holmes *et al.* (2002); Ballard *et al.* (2002)
Music therapy: includes playing and/or listening to music as a way of generally enhancing well-being. Can be used in movement therapies.	A Cochrane review by Vink and Birks (2009) identified five studies. However, the quality of the studies were poor. As such, the reviewers concluded there was insufficient evidence to view the approach as effective.	Lord and Garner (1993); Gotell *et al.* (2002)

Intervention	Evidence	References
Environmental manipulation: use of environmental cues, signage and appropriate building layout in order to facilitate communication, exercise and pleasure and to reduce disorientation.	A Cochrane review by Forbes *et al.* 2009 on the use of bright light therapy in terms of mood, sleep and behaviour reviewed three trials. However, the quality of the studies was poor. As such, the reviewers concluded there was insufficient evidence to view the approach as effective. A Cochrane review by Price *et al.* (2001 updated 2009) on the use of environmental and social barriers to prevent wandering failed to identify suitable trails.	Judd, Marshall and Phippen (1997); Day *et al.* (2000)
II Formulation-led approaches		
Behavioural management techniques: based on learning theory and utilising the antecedents and consequences of behaviour to devise and execute interventions.	A systematic review by Spira and Edelstein (2006) reported 23 studies. These tended to be of poor to moderate quality, and many were single case design. Moniz-Cook *et al.* are currently undertaking a Cochrane review to be published 2011.	Moniz-Cook *et al.* (in press)
Psychotherapies: the use of cognitive behavioural therapy, interpersonal psychotherapy and other standard psychotherapeutic formats. Used with patients in early stages of dementia.	NICE (2004) guidelines for depression recommend both CBT and IPT in the treatment of moderate depression. Teri *et al.* (1997) demonstrated the positive impact of CBT on mood and problem-solving abilities in people with dementia.	Teri *et al.* (1991); Miller and Reynolds (2002); Miller (2008)

In the following sections, psychological approaches will be described in some detail and further information included on their evidence-base. The discussions will include findings from controlled and non-controlled studies. As one will see, when permitting the inclusion of poorer quality studies, more therapies become available to discuss although the evidence-base supporting them becomes correspondingly weaker. Before discussing the approaches it is worth noting the importance of matching the methods to the cognitive and physical abilities of the person with dementia; a number of the occupational therapy programmes place particular emphasis on this aspect (Perrin and May 2000). They identify and exploit preserved abilities (e.g. procedural, over-learned memories – e.g. abilities to play instruments, dance, knit, etc.), in helping the person to remain active and achieve a high level of well-being.

PSYCHOLOGICAL APPROACHES: PREVENTION VERSUS INTERVENTION

There are many psychological therapies used in the treatment of challenging behaviours. Hulme *et al.* (2010) present a systematic review of previous reviews of such treatments. They identify 33 articles, which describe 13 types of intervention: animal assisted, aromatherapy, CST, environmental, light, massage, music, physical activity, Reality Orientation, reminiscence, multi-sensory, validation and electrical nerve stimulation (TENS). The therapies have been used in a preventative capacity, where carers intentionally engage in activities to reduce the client's levels of distress, depression and agitation and thereby reducing the likelihood of a BC emerging. Indeed, it is suggested that improving people's general levels of contentment prevents the emergence of an 'unmet' need. Figure 4.3 outlines some of the themes associated with high levels of well-being in dementia. However, once a BC has emerged a more intensive, intervention strategy is called for. In the latter case the strategies selected would be tailored to the specific needs of the individual in relation to the problematic behaviour. It is important to recognise that the rationales are different, with the intervention strategies normally being guided by a formulation.

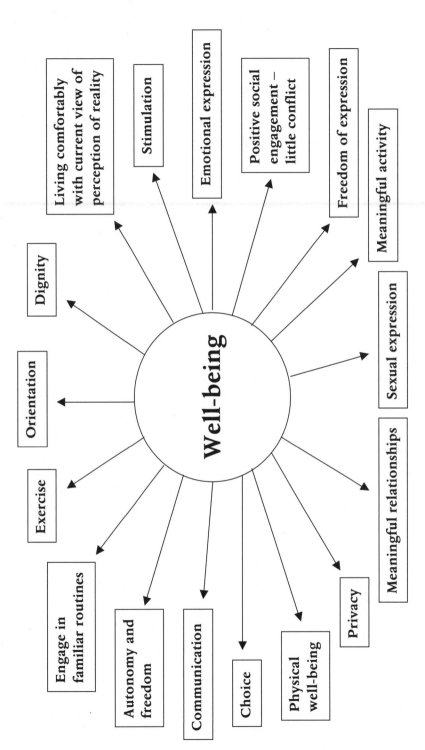

Figure 4.3 Themes associated with well-being

In the following section, preventative therapies will be discussed, both the mainstream approaches and some 'alternatives' (e.g. music therapy, dance, aromatherapy, animal assisted activities). In the second section information about interventions strategies will be presented.

Mainstream preventative strategies
Reality orientation (RO)

This approach attempts to orientate patients with dementia to the 'present' via the use of cues (clocks, calendars, newspapers) and/or discussion. The rationale underpinning this strategy suggests that owing to memory and orientation problems, people with dementia are often confused and this may lead to social disengagement. However, if one is able to provide cues that enable them to engage in what is happening in the 'here and now', they are able to participate in social interactions in a more confident and fulfilling way. The provision of environmental cues (e.g. signs, picture boards) also has the advantage of assisting people to find their way around their setting. When using this approach it is essential that one employs it sensitively, ensuring people are re-orientated in a validating way. There is debate regarding the efficacy of the approach (Verkaik *et al.* 2005), even in light of Spector *et al.*'s (2002a) favourable Cochrane review of six randomised controlled trials (RCTs). The debate centres around claims that RO can remind the participants of their deterioration (Goudie and Stokes 1989), and also lead to repeated confrontations with the person with dementia. For example, someone, who mistakenly thinks he is 30 and still working as a miner may become upset when orientated to the reality of his current situation (however sensitively done!).

Cognitive stimulation therapy (CST)

CST involves activating people's remaining cognitive functioning through the presentation of stimulating information (e.g. use of physical games; word and number games; everyday objects – see Spector *et al.* 2006). Recent studies show promise for this approach for people with mild to moderate dementia (NICE 2006), and also demonstrate its cost effectiveness due to the fact that it can often be performed in a group setting (Knapp *et al.* 2006). In Spector's programmes, the members of the group typically attend 7 weeks, twice weekly sessions each lasting 45 minutes. The foci of the sessions are diverse themes, such as discussions about food, childhood, significant memories, etc. In comparison to a control group, those attending CST show improvements in cognition and quality of life. Livingston *et al.*'s (2005) recent systematic review of six studies of various quality (e.g. Spector *et al.* 2003; Romero and Wenz 2001) concluded that this approach consistently showed promise across a range of situations. This view has been confirmed in the latest Cochrane review (Woods *et al.* 2009). Currently, there is a great deal of ongoing work examining the long-term effects of CST, patient acceptability, and the mechanisms of change associated with it. Much of this work is taking place under the SHIELD research programme (Support at Home Interventions to Enhance Life in Dementia).

Reminiscence therapy (RMT)

RMT involves people reliving past experiences, especially those that might be positive and personally significant, such as family holidays or weddings. This therapy can be used as a group therapy or with individuals. Group sessions employ activities such as art, music and often use artefacts to provide cues and stimulation. RMT is seen as a way of increasing levels of well-being, providing pleasure and cognitive stimulation. When working with people with dementia, care staff and families are often encouraged to jointly construct historical reviews of the residents' lives (i.e. life stories). Life story work is helpful in promoting attachments between staff and residents, particularly in cases where residents have poor communication skills. There is growing evidence that RMT is an effective treatment for older people with and without dementia (see Woods *et al.* 2005b and Bohlmeijer *et al.* 2003 respectively). On the whole, the approach has many supporters (Warner *et al.* 2006; Verkaik *et al.* 2005) due to its flexibility and adaptability to the individual's needs (e.g. a person with severe dementia can still gain pleasure from listening to a favourite old record). It is relevant to note that the approach needs to be used carefully because many people have undergone difficult times in their pasts (losses, abuse, mental illness, etc.), and reactivating such memories can have negative consequences. In my clinical work, I refer to the inadvertent recall of negative memories as 're-infection'. Once a problematic event has been retrieved it may be particularly difficult to cope with (i.e. resolve, repress, etc.) because of the person's cognitive deficits (James 2010).

Validation therapy (VT)

It is suggested that some of the features associated with dementia, such as repetition of past events and stories, are active strategies to avoid stress, boredom and loneliness. Naomi Feil argues that people with dementia can retreat into an inner reality based on 'feelings' rather than 'intellect', as they find their present reality too painful (Feil and Klerk-Rubin 2002). VT therapists thus attempt to communicate with the person with dementia through empathising with the feelings and hidden meanings behind their confused speech and behaviour. It is the emotional content of what is being said that is therefore more important than the person's orientation to the present. Neal and Barton Wright's (2003) Cochrane review evaluated VT's effectiveness across a number of controlled trials, employing cognitive and behavioural measures (Finnema *et al.* 2005). They concluded that despite some positive indicators in terms of depression (Toseland *et al.* 1997), the jury was still out with respect to its effectiveness.

Psychomotor therapy

Psychomotor therapy, sometimes referred to as activity therapy, is a rather varied group of action-based activities, such as dance, sport, drama, etc. A recent study by Cohen-Mansfield and her colleagues (Cohen-Mansfield *et al.* 2010) demonstrated the positive impact of a range of such activities for residents in care. In her study she monitored the impact of 25 different tasks undertaken over a three week period (i.e. conversations, interactions with animals, use of toys, reading, listening to music, folding towels, flower arranging, puzzles, artistic activities, etc.). For each of the activities both the amount of perceived enjoyment obtained from the task and the length of 'time spent' engaging in the task were assessed. The findings revealed that the most enjoyable tasks were those that involved engaging with living things (people, real baby, animals), followed by tasks involving some form of social simulation (use of dolls, simulation presence videos, etc). However, when length of engagement was assessed (i.e. length of time spent on task), the residents spent longer on tasks that mimicked work-like activities (stamping envelopes, sorting jewellery, folding towels). These results are likely to have important consequences in terms of the sorts of activities one might suggest to carers to help occupy people with dementia in order to enhance well-being, increase self-worth and relieve boredom. It has been shown that physical exercise can have a number of health benefits for older people, including those in care settings (Heyn *et al.* 2004; Eggermont and Scherder 2006). Positive effects have occurred in terms of reductions in falls, improvements in mental health and sleep (King *et al.* 1997; Winstead-Fry and Kijek 1999), and also an increase in older people's mood and confidence (Singh *et al.* 2005). In addition, Alessi *et al.* (1999) found in a small-scale controlled study that daytime exercise helped to reduce daytime agitation and night-time restlessness (Montgomery and Dennis 2002). Despite these findings, two of the three better quality controlled trials conducted in the area failed to find significant differences in terms of depression and apathy when compared to 'normal' care (Hopman-Rock *et al.* 1999). In Newcastle, Guzman-Garcia, a PhD student, has been investigating the use of Latin American Dancing by care home residents. The pilot studies have demonstrated benefits for both people with dementia and their carers. Figure 4.4 shows some of the key benefits reported by staff (Guzman-Garcia, James and Mukaetova-Ladinska, in press).

Multi-sensory therapy

Up and down the country there are care homes and wards that have invested in multi-sensory rooms. The typical equipment within such rooms includes: coloured lights, fibre optic tubes, bubble columns, music systems, etc., all of which are designed to stimulate people's senses (Baker *et al.* 2001). Unfortunately, a lack of training in the use of the facilities, means that often the rooms are under-utilised, and even sometimes avoided by staff and residents. In most circumstances, the use of multi-sensory therapy should be tailored to the needs of each individual; therefore all of the methods of stimulation (use of auditory stimuli, lights, textures) may not necessarily be used in one session (Chung and Lai 2002). A Cochrane report of this therapy stated that overall the findings were, as yet, inconclusive (Chung and Lai 2008). However, more recently, Verkaik *et al.*'s (2005) review has suggested that multi-sensory approaches may be effective in the treatment of apathy and depression both in care settings and in the community.

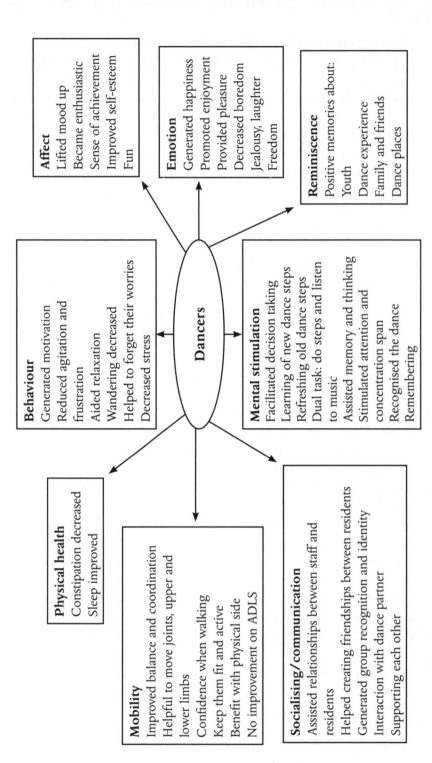

Affect
Lifted mood up
Became enthusiastic
Sense of achievement
Improved self-esteem
Fun

Emotion
Generated happiness
Promoted enjoyment
Provided pleasure
Decreased boredom
Jealousy, laughter
Freedom

Reminiscence
Positive memories about:
Youth
Dance experience
Family and friends
Dance places

Behaviour
Generated motivation
Reduced agitation and
frustration
Aided relaxation
Wandering decreased
Helped to forget their worries
Decreased stress

Dancers

Mental stimulation
Facilitated decision taking
Learning of new dance steps
Refreshing old dance steps
Dual task: do steps and listen
to music
Assisted memory and thinking
Stimulated attention and
concentration span
Recognised the dance
Remembering

Physical health
Constipation decreased
Sleep improved

Mobility
Improved balance and coordination
Helpful to move joints, upper and
lower limbs
Confidence when walking
Keep them fit and active
Benefit with physical side
No improvement on ADLS

Socialising/communication
Assisted relationships between staff and
residents
Helped creating friendships between residents
Generated group recognition and identity
Interaction with dance partner
Supporting each other

Figure 4.4 Benefits of dance psychomotor therapy (Guzman-Garcia et al. in press)

Alternative preventative psychological strategies
Aromatherapy
The two main essential oils used in aromatherapy for dementia are extracted from lavender and lemon balm. There have been positive results from recent controlled trials that have shown significant improvements in agitation symptoms with excellent compliance and tolerability (Holmes *et al.* 2002; Ballard *et al.* 2002). It is relevant to note, however, that Thorgrimsen *et al.*'s (2003) review stated that there were flaws in both of these controlled studies, and thus the findings must be treated with caution. Of note, the latest review examining aromatherapy has revealed mixed findings, describing its efficacy as 'scarce' (Quynh-anh and Paton 2008). The article also called upon future researchers to examine the potential side-effects of the treatment.

Music therapy
The poor quality of studies on this topic has been noted in the Cochrane review (Vink and Birks 2009). Nevertheless, it has long been accepted within the scientific literature that music can have a profound effect on people's mood and well-being (Sherrat *et al.* 2004). Indeed, music is used as a mood-inducing technique in a number of clinical trials, where the music produces a state that temporarily induces depression (Clark 1983). Music is also considered useful in reducing unwanted behaviour, and improving communication, particularly when tailored to people's taste. For example, Lord and Garner (1993) showed increased levels of well-being, better social skills and improvements in autobiographical memory in a group of residents interacting with bespoke music. Such improvements were not observed in a comparison group engaged in other activities. Music has also been shown to reduce agitation at meal times, assisting people to remain seated for longer at their tables (Chang *et al.* 2005). There have also been reported improvements in depressive symptoms through participation in reminiscence focused music groups (Ashida 2002), and improvements in communication and irritability when engaged in structured playing of music (Suzuki *et al.* 2004). As with all strategies, care needs to be used when using this approach because music can cue problematic memories too. For example, I recall a person whose screaming was eventually found be related to the playing of 1940s 'war-time' music at the day centre. From examining her history, we found this period of her life was taxing. She lost most of her family and had experienced abuse as an evacuee.

Art therapy

Art therapy (drama, model making, drawing and painting) is a treatment in which people have the opportunity to explore new skills (Mottram 2003) and thereby enhance their self-esteem. In the case of people with dementia, art therapy has been shown to provide meaningful stimulation, and improve social interaction and levels of self-esteem (Killick and Allan 1999). One of the few quality studies in the area was a controlled study investigating the effects of drama and movement on depression in groups of day-hospital attendees (Wilkinson *et al.* 1998). Despite some favourable indicators, no significant findings were observed in terms of depression compared to those receiving routine care.

Animal assisted activities

Animals introduced into nursing homes as regular visitors or as home-pets have been shown to have positive effects, including reducing blood pressure, agitation, strain, tension, loneliness and increasing life expectancy (Churchill *et al.* 1999; Richeson 2003). Short-term interactions with dogs have been shown to increase social interaction with, and between, older people with mental impairment (Greer *et al.* 2001). The presence of other types of animal have also demonstrated benefits. For example, the use of a fish tank in a dining area has been shown to reduce aggression and enhance the nutritional intake of home residents with dementia (Edwards 2004). Before introducing animals into care settings, the relevant authorities need to be contacted due to health and safety requirements and matters to do with infection control.

Using dolls and toys

The use of dolls and toys in care settings is not new (Libin and Cohen-Mansfield 2004), but has only recently been studied in a systematic manner (James *et al.* 2005; Mackenzie *et al.* 2006). Investigations have involved the introduction of dolls and teddy bears into care homes following a standard format (Mackenzie *et al.* 2006). Typically, staff are given information and guidelines on their use prior to their introduction (Mackenzie *et al.* 2007). The findings from these investigations have been favourable for both residents and staff (Mackenzie *et al.* 2006; James *et al.* 2006a – see Chapter 8). This approach is clearly controversial and an ongoing debate within the *Journal of Dementia Care* (Wood-Mitchell *et al.* 2006, 2007a) has demonstrated resistance to the technique as it can be viewed as 'patronising' and promoting 'infantilisation'. In response to such arguments, a Teesside University doctorate student is currently collecting information from people with dementia, examining their views on the use of dolls (Alander *et al.* 2010).

Tool-box approaches

Some of the above strategies have been presented as stand-alone techniques, but it is evident that often carers combine them and use them in non-standard ways. A good example of this is the various forms of 'tool-box' techniques (Thwaites and Sara 2010). This widely used approach involves creating an individualised box of items for each person, containing personalised material (e.g. photographs, postcards, camcorder recordings of family scenes or voices, items of clothes, ornaments, relevant maps, aromatherapy oils). The staff can use the items in the box to stimulate and communicate with the individual, learning more about the person's history and promoting positive reminiscence. In our own clinics we have found the simulated presence items (using recordings of family and friends) to be effective in reducing agitation.

In addition to the approaches outlined above there are a number of multi-activity programmes specifically designed to promote well-being. Two well-established examples of this are SPECAL and SONAS apc. The SPECAL approach (Specialized Elderly Care for Alzheimer and Dementia, Garner 2004) uses people's preserved memories (verbal and behavioural) to improve and maintain their moods: 'A person with dementia will experience random, intermittent and increasingly frequent memory blanks relating to recent events. However, in practically all cases, some memories of past events remain securely stored and can be readily recalled by the person, given the right circumstances' (www. specal.co.uk). Via the SPECAL approach carers are provided with an explanation of what dementia might be like to live with, for the person with dementia. It uses the analogy of a photograph album to represent how memory works, that is, this explanation underpins all principles and is central to the development of a number of memory-based therapeutic approaches (e.g. helping people to utilise life-long skills and re-engage in interests).

The SONAS apc approach (Threadgold 2002) is based on stimulation of the senses, structure and repetition, and is focused on communication. Group and individual sessions are recorded on a CD to enable those carrying out the sessions to focus completely on the participants. The group sessions involve stimulation of all five senses, music, singalongs, gentle movement, memory-focused exercises and a time for personal contributions. Trained facilitators carry out the sessions with about eight participants. Repetition builds familiarity and security for the participants. The focus on abilities rather than disabilities and the creation of a failure-free environment create an atmosphere in which people are free to express themselves without judgement (Moriaty *et al.* 2003).

Before completing this section it is important to acknowledge the work of the Bradford group and their development of dementia care mapping (DCM, Kitwood and Bredin 1992). Although not a therapy in itself, it is a system that monitors people's well-being over time, and it provides carers with feedback about their communication style. Dementia care mapping has been shown to be a highly effective clinical and training tool, and has been customised for organisations and assessors (Brooker 2006).

Within the DCM approach, training the carers is seen as a key feature. Indeed, many of the above approaches are ineffective, and potentially harmful, if not conducted well. On a positive note, most of the approaches described above are accompanied by published guidelines that describe how to use them appropriately and sensitively (Brooker 2007).

Intervention strategies

In the following section a number of 'formulation-led' approaches are described. Here, typically a BC has already been observed (hitting, shouting, etc.) and the intervention procedure is specifically targeted at its causes. These interventions routinely involve the development of a formulation (i.e. a descriptive account of the BC in relation to the person and her past) to help understand the triggering and maintaining features of the problem (Cohen-Mansfield *et al.* 2007). First some standard psychotherapeutic approaches will be described (cognitive behaviour therapy [CBT]; interpersonal therapy [IPT]), whose use is limited to those with mild impairment (James 2010). I will then go on to discuss therapies that can be used with all presentations, even with cases of severe dementia (behaviour therapy and needs-led frameworks). It is relevant to note that the function of the formulation of the standard psychotherapies differs with that of the two latter therapies. For example, CBT and IPT formulations are designed to aid 'clients' gain a better understanding of their problems; this requires the clients to have a degree of insight into their difficulties and the abilities to initiate change with respect to their behaviour. In contrast, behaviour therapy (BT) and the needs-led frameworks employ formulations as vehicles to enable carers to gain a better understanding of the difficulties of people with dementia. This is particularly important because in cases of severe dementia, it is the carers who are required to carry out the interventions.

Standard psychotherapies

Over the last ten years there has been an increasing interest in applying CBT and IPT to people with cognitive impairment (James 2010; Miller and Reynolds 2007). In relation to BC, these therapies are used in cases of low mood, anxiety or when the person with dementia retains insight and problem-solving abilities. CBT examines people's distress within a cycle (see Figure 4.5a and b); in order to alter the inner feeling, the outer features are worked on. The cognitive aspects (i.e. thoughts and beliefs) receive particular attention, because when people are distressed, they tend to engage in negative thinking (e.g. I am worthless; Everyone hates me; No-one wants me, etc.). CBT has developed strategies to help people re-evaluate their thinking, and to start re-engaging in 'helpful' activities and relationships they have been avoiding (James 2010).

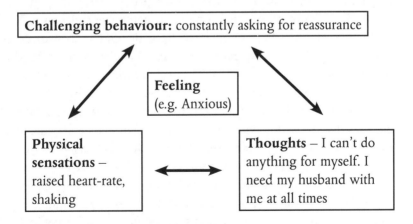

Figure 4.5 a) Triad for someone with a mild dementia

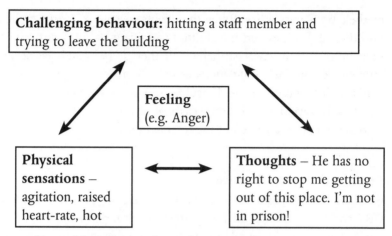

Figure 4.5 b) Triad for someone with a moderate-severe dementia

It is relevant to note that this triad is also helpful in understanding the problematic behaviour of those with more severe dementia (see Figure 4.5b), with their behaviours linked to their distorted sense of their current reality. However, their neurological deficits prevent them being able to make changes for themselves.

Teri and Gallagher-Thompson (1991) reported positive findings from a clinical trial of CBT with people in the early stages of Alzheimer's disease. Single case and group CBT have also been used by other researchers with some favourable results (Koder 1998; Kipling *et al.* 1999). It is worth noting that a number of the principles of CBT are embedded in the service-model we have devised in Newcastle (see Chapter 6), and it is transparent that these principles form the backbone of our work with carers and staff (James, Powell and Kendell 2001). These issues are discussed in detail in the next two chapters.

Interpersonal therapy (IPT), as the name suggests, examines the person's distress within an interpersonal context. People are encouraged to look at how important relationships have changed since they have become distressed, and they are also asked to examine their communication-styles to see if it can be improved. Such an approach is particularly relevant for those therapists who see BC as a 'communication strategy in a form other people find socially unacceptable'. For example, a person with poor verbal skills and reduced insight is unable to ask for food, and so he takes it from someone else. There is some overlap of IPT with the person-centred work of Kitwood (1997) and Stokes (2001). There is good empirical evidence for this form of treatment with older people (Miller and Reynolds 2002); it has only recently been applied in the area of dementia (James 2010; James *et al.* 2003a; Miller and Reynolds 2007). Owing to the demands IPT places on insightfulness and the ability to reflect, its use remains rather limited in the treatment of people with moderate to severe dementia.

Carer-centred, person-focused approaches

The following approaches can be employed for a range of clinical presentations, even in situations where clients have either poor communication skills and/or poor insight; thus these methods are suitable for working with people with severe dementia. The key reason they can be employed with this group is that although the focus of the treatment is directed at the person with dementia, much of the actual work is done via carers. Due to this, working with these interventions requires a systems approach, whereby much of the success depends on supporting the carers to deliver the therapy effectively. For this reason, the approaches are termed 'carer-centred, person-focused'.

Behaviour therapy (BT)

Behaviour therapy requires a detailed assessment period in which the triggers, behaviours and reinforcers (i.e. the antecedents, behaviour and consequences – ABC) are identified and their relationships made clear. This process is frequently referred to as a Functional Assessment (Moniz-Cook *et al.* 2001a, in press). The therapist will often use some kind of chart or diary to gather information about the manifestations of a behaviour (B) and the sequence of actions leading up to it (A). The reactions to the behaviour (C) are also studied because they frequently serve to either increase or decrease the likelihood of the action occurring again. Such monitoring helps to identify the BC's function, and the accurate observations are essential in generating better hypotheses. For example, consider the case of Joan, whose continual shouting was initially attributed to arthritic pain. However, the functional assessment revealed that she only shouted in the presence of men. This meant her pain killers could be stopped, which relieved her constipation, and the new data allowed the therapist to focus on her issues with men, enabling her therapists to go on to develop a more appropriate intervention.

Teri *et al.* (1997) developed and conducted an 11-session training programme to teach 41 carers of individuals with dementia how to manage agitated behaviour using functional analysis based behavioural interventions in their home environment. During sessions carers worked with a therapist to define problem behaviours, complete and interpret functional analyses, and develop interventions. Teri *et al.* (1998) presented four case studies to illustrate the effectiveness of their programme. The antecedents to the four participants' agitation were found to be: (a) lack of activity; (b) confrontation over confused statements; (c) inactivity specifically at dusk; and (d) lack of social attention due to caregiver completing tasks, respectively. Consequently antecedent control interventions were designed (e.g. providing appropriately tailored activities).

For one participant the interventions resulted in the elimination of verbal and physical aggression. For the other three participants reductions in agitated and aggressive behaviours were found. Unfortunately no data were presented and limited qualitative feedback from the participants were reported as outcome measures, making it difficult to interpret how successful the interventions actually were.

The efficacy of BT has been demonstrated in the context of dementia in a number of studies (Doyle *et al.* 1997; Allen-Burge *et al.* 1999; Fossey *et al.* 2006). Spira and Edelstein (2006) have recently undertaken a systematic review of the use of BT with people with dementia and reported optimistic findings. However, they noted that few of the 23 articles that met their inclusion criteria could be regarded as 'quality' studies. A more rigorous Cochrane review has been conducted by Moniz-Cook *et al.* (in press). She identified 15 trials, ten from family care settings and five from residential care settings. For the primary outcome of frequency of problematic behaviours, only ten studies (n = 1140 participants) had usable data. She concluded that whilst FA showed promise, it is too early to provide an indication of its effectiveness. This is because the evidence rests largely on a handful of studies for which its actual effects are unclear, since the intervention tended to be delivered within broad multi-component programmes of psychosocial interventions. Furthermore the studies were generally small and the duration of interventions varied across studies.

Needs-led therapies

Currently there are a number of conceptual models that examine BC in terms of people's needs (Cohen-Mansfield 2000b; James 1999; James *et al.* 2006b). These frameworks typically involve obtaining two types of information: (i) background features (history, premorbid personality and coping style, cognitive status, mental health status, physical health status, environmental and contextual status) and (ii) a comprehensive description of the BC episode – a functional assessment. By putting these two types of information together, one is in a stronger position to accurately identify the person's needs. The needs-based models highlight the fact that BC are usually not unpredictable random actions, rather they are rational activities with a high degree of predictability. Indeed, frequently BC are manifestations of residents' attempts to fulfil an unmet need. For example:

- BC as a method of trying to achieve a need (e.g. Breaking a window in order to get outside of the care facility and walk in the garden).

- BC as a means of fulfilling one's need (e.g. Urinating in a sink in order to relieve the pressure in one's bladder).

- BC as an expression of frustration that a need is not being met (e.g. Hitting a member of staff who is insisting you go to bed when you are enjoying a late night TV programme).

Cohen-Mansfield (2000a,b) provides one of the best descriptions of an unmet needs model, and her recent empirical study testifies to the efficacy of her approach (Cohen-Mansfield *et al.* 2007). The fundamentals of her work are based on Maslow's hierarchy of needs: the need for physiological/physical well-being; safety; love and belonging; esteem; self-actualisation. She believes that BC often occur when the 'vulnerable and disadvantaged' person strives to have some of these fundamental needs met. She believes that such striving is often problematic for people with dementia because of the following difficulties: poor communication; inability to use their prior coping mechanisms; unable to meet their own needs without the assistance of others. There are often additional difficulties because the person's environment may not be able to provide the 'need', or the setting may simply not understand it. As with the Newcastle model (James and Stephenson 2007), Cohen-Mansfield places a great emphasis on tailoring her treatment for each individual.

Bird *et al.* (2007) are also exponents of the needs-led perspective, and have provided numerous case-examples of the benefits of his methodology. More recently Bird has undertaken a controlled-study that illustrates the efficacy of his work (Bird *et al.* 2009). In Chapters 6 and 7 the needs-led methodology used by the NCBT is outlined. In Chapter 7 a number of case examples will be used to illustrate this methodology, which is termed a 'carer-centred person-focused' approach. Within the Newcastle team we have developed a number of guides to help us work well with carers, and these have become operating principles for members of the team. One of these helpful guidelines is termed LCAPS (see Table 4.2). The acronym LCAPS refers to the following steps: Listen, Clarify, Agree, Plan, Support.

The LCAPS features remind us that it is the carers who provide the majority of the input, and who assist the person in meeting her need, and therefore it is vital the carers are listened to, respected, and guided. Indeed, the carers need to have their say, be provided with additional information, be guided to some hypotheses, and to be inspired to exchange current practices for new ones based on a sensible and practical rationale. A practical example of how this can be done is provided in Chapter 6, within the description of the Newcastle Model. In Chapter 6 the therapeutic skills required to deliver a 'needs-led' approach are discussed, particularly the questioning skills required of the therapist.

CONCLUSION

I am often asked by managers, 'What is an effective psychological approach for challenging behaviour?' and the questioners get frustrated when I respond, 'It depends on who is doing what, how, when and where.' Evidently, some managers want a 'magic bullet', a psychological equivalent to a highly effective tablet. Unfortunately, there is no such therapy or product that we can draw upon. Rather, owing to the multi-factorial causes of BC, it is usually necessary to undertake a careful assessment and develop a formulated and personally tailored intervention from this (Vernooij-Dassen *et al.* 2010).

This chapter has also demonstrated that BC work is not always about being reactive. For example, the chapter has outlined a number of proactive, preventative strategies designed to reduce the likelihood of BC emerging in the first place. Thus one would expect that in those settings seeking to promote clients' well-being, carers would be using both the preventative and intervention strategies.

Table 4.2 LCAPS guidelines for working with care staff

	Principle	Features involved
Listen	The therapist needs to listen to the various stories relating to the CB from those being affected by the behaviour. He needs to investigate what strategies have been tried before, and how successful they were.	It is important that those affected are allowed to give their views on why the behaviour is happening. This may be the first time they've had the opportunity to give their views, and it is good for them to hear themselves articulating their story; this can produce change in itself. Relevant beliefs and emotions are noted. The therapist's role is to listen and not challenge too much at this stage. Background information is also collected which helps to put the behaviour in context. A record of previously tried strategies is helpful in order to see what was successful in the past, including information about who related best to the person with dementia.
Clarify	The stories provided need to be checked out and clarified because they often contain contradictory information. The facts of the situation need to be clarified (e.g. What is the behaviour, when it occurs, when not occurring, who is present, etc.)	The therapist armed with the background information, and his knowledge of both dementia and CBs starts to check-out some of the inconsistencies in the various stories. His role is also to start imparting relevant information, and to distinguish the facts of the situation from any 'unsupported' assumptions. Another task is to discriminate between the emotionally-based thinking from the factually-based evidence. As part of this clarification process, the therapist will investigate what things seemed to have worked previously, and why they were not working now. And also who was best at relating to the person with dementia, and what could be learned from the style of this carer.

Table 4.2 LCAPS guidelines for working with care staff cont.

	Principle	Features involved
Agree	The therapist much achieve an agreed, unifying version of story that provides possible solutions.	Having assessed the situation, the next step is to produce a single version (story) regarding the behaviour. This normally involves organising a meeting with all those involved in order to get mutually acceptable version of events.
Plan	The therapist must develop a treatment strategy collaboratively with the person and carers to deal with the problematic situation.	The mutually agreed story provides the platform from which treatment strategies are developed. These strategies also need to be agreed in the presence of everyone in order that the treatment rationale and aims can be clarified and agreed respectively.
Support	The therapist should support the implementation of the treatment strategy.	If a new treatment approach has been devised, it will often require guidance, modelling, etc. to facilitate implementation. In some circumstances no particular strategy is deemed appropriate, and thus people may require support to enable them to tolerate the ongoing behaviour better.

Chapter 5

Conceptual Models Used to Aid Assessment and Treatment

INTRODUCTION

Throughout this book it has been noted that there is a poor evidence-base regarding the effectiveness of many of the non-pharmacological therapies. From my perspective, I feel a hindrance to establishing their credentials has been the lack of theories regarding people's experiences of dementia. There are relatively few exceptions to this, most of which are discussed in the following chapter (e.g. Cohen-Mansfield 2000a; Kitwood 1997; Stokes 2001, etc.). If we contrast this impoverished position with that of treatments for the affective disorders, we can see that the various theoretical models derived for depression, panic, obsessive-compulsive disorder, psychosis, etc., have enabled the development of tailored treatment packages; each with its own evidence-base (James 2010). Further, because the latter disorders have frameworks that show how distress is derived and maintained, clinical insight is gained in how the distress can be alleviated.

This chapter presents a number of conceptual models for dementia and BC. The goal of this work is to provide a set of frameworks around which successful interventions can be developed. Having presented the models, the reader will be in a position to choose which one is most appropriate to use in a given situation.

By the end of this chapter the reader will be aware of the following:

- There are a number of conceptual models which provide insight into the distress experienced by people with dementia.

- The models can assist therapists in conducting assessments and guiding their interventions.

- It is often useful to conceptualise the dynamics occurring between the person with dementia and the carer in order to facilitate empathy and to provide a platform for change.

CONCEPTUAL MODELS

Conceptual models are valued in the therapy literature because they provide structure, giving guidance on what to assess and how to intervene (James 2010; Volicer and Hurley 2003). They also allow the development of clearer rationales regarding treatment approaches. For example, if one's model shows there to be four key aspects maintaining a problem, a considered decision can be made about which one is best to tackle first. One could also predict the possible knock-on effects of tackling one issue in relation to the other features in the model. For example, if a person's aggression is seen to be a product of feeling anxious and vulnerable, it would make sense to treat the anxiety in order to eliminate the aggression. This chapter examines several conceptual models within three broad groups. The first group considers those models used to conceptualise the experience of dementia, using rather generic frameworks. This is followed by a section which discusses the models that are more specific to BC and its treatment (p.91). Finally, there is a section which presents a model that describes the emotional dynamics that can occur between people with dementia and their carers (p.98).

Conceptualisations of dementia
Kitwood's five elements model (1997)
Kitwood's simple linear and descriptive formulation uses five features to help therapists understand a client's experience of dementia. The assessment requires the therapist to collect details about the person's: premorbid personality + history + health status + intellectual impairment + environment. Although not a sophisticated model, it requires the

therapist to look beyond the medical aspects of the disease and pay attention to the person and her history. For example, knowing the person had children can help us understand why she frequently asks to leave the ward at 5 pm when she sees school children pass the window of her care home.

While this model is helpful, Kitwood's framework is descriptive rather than explanatory, and thus is not a good guide for interventions. A rather more informative model is the conceptualisation of dementia (CoD) framework. This model attempts to describe some of the processes occurring for people with dementia, which may lead them to become depressed, anxious, and/or aggressive.

Conceptualisation of dementia (CoD) framework (James 2010)

Figure 5.1 presents the CoD framework diagrammatically; it is essentially an ABC model (Events, Reactions, Consequences). The experiencing of the event is influenced by the person with dementia's thoughts and attitudes. The 'perception of self' aspect is determined by the contextual factors to do with the individual's premorbid personality, history, and cognitive status. Indeed, the person's prior social status, personality type, previous job, life-roles, religious and sexual preferences, physical status, fears, responses to illness, etc. will all influence the way she views herself during the various stages of the dementing process.

In the early stages of the illness, when the level of insight remains high, the person will be aware she is having memory and processing difficulties and may take this into account in her reactions to events. For example, because she is aware she keeps forgetting whether she's taken her tablets, she is less inclined to argue with her husband when told she's forgotten her medication. In situations that result in negative consequences, (e.g. she gets repeatedly criticised or lost), her confidence may become undermined, and she may start to feel anxious, shameful or low.

As the person begins to lose insight, and her sense of reality becomes less similar to others, interactions with her environment may become more problematic ('A'). This may evoke a range of negative emotions and coping strategies. Some of these strategies ('B' – reassurance seeking, avoidance, etc.) may be viewed as challenging within the environment she is living in (own home, sheltered accommodation, hospital, care home, etc.). The environment's response (i.e. the physical and social Consequences – 'C')

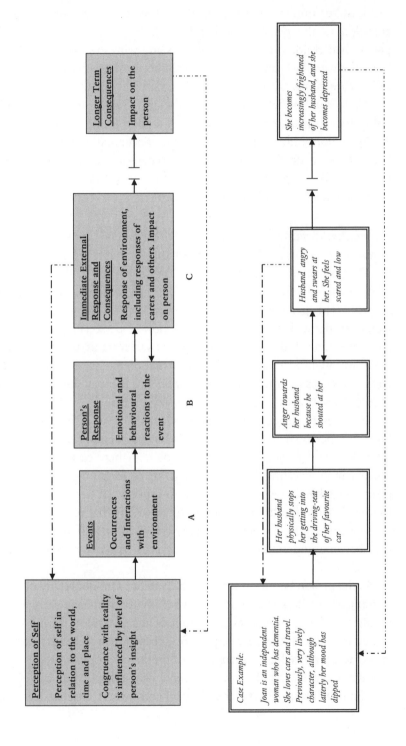

Figure 5.1 Conceptualisation of dementia (CoD)

to her reactions can evoke further emotional and behavioural reactions, leading to 'challenging behaviours'. As an example, consider a 89-year-old resident who does not believe her keyworker when told she can't leave the care-home to collect her 'young' children from their school. The woman could very easily become aggressive if orientated to the facts in an non-empathic manner; particularly if the carer fails to take account of the woman's incorrect perception of reality. Of note, her response may be more positive if spoken to in a way that accommodates her own sense of reality, for example, via the use of validation techniques (Feil and de Klerk-Rubin 2002).

The longer term consequence of such occurrences will have a cumulative impact on the person's self-esteem. For example, if the response of the environment is routinely punitive or hostile, the person may develop a sense of mistrust, learned helplessness, or unworthiness. If this is the routine experience, the person may become depressed.

While this model is helpful in understanding how negative information can feed into making the person feel worse, it is also useful as a means of promoting well-being. Indeed, it highlights the need to understand the person's level of insight and current perception of self. It also calls upon therapists to interact with the client in ways that promote a positive self-perspective.

The value of the CoD model is that it not only outlines some of the key features relating to people's experiences, it also looks at the processes involved in producing them. Therefore by altering features occurring at each of the stages in the diagram, it suggests we are able to influence whether things are going to be made worse or better for the person with dementia. For example, in the case outlined in Figure 5.1, if the husband had not sworn at his wife when she became angry, she would not have become frightened of him, etc. Further, if we were able to support him in responding more empathically rather than aggressively, we may have been able to improve her self-esteem.

The next section examines models designed to provide better insight into factors associated with BC.

Conceptual models for challenging behaviour

The following six frameworks address issues associated with BC. However, they have differing functions. Stokes (2001) emphasises the importance of seeing the 'person' rather than merely the dementia. The second, third and fourth models (Kunik *et al.* 2003; Volicer and Hurley 2003; Cohen-Mansfield 2000a) are all frameworks for guiding assessments and interventions. Of note, the fifth model, Cohen-Mansfield's unmet need perspective, is currently the best known conceptualisation for BC. The final model is the one we have developed in Newcastle. It integrates features of the other frameworks, and forms the basis of the clinical formulations used by the Newcastle Challenging Behaviour Team (NCBT), which are illustrated in Chapter 6 and 7.

Stokes' psychogenic model of challenging behaviour (Stokes 2001)

Stokes' model (see Figure 5.2) highlights that once someone is diagnosed with dementia other people tend to attribute the causes of her problems to the disease, paying less attention to the psychological aspects. Thus if someone with dementia is aggressive when being escorted to the toilet the cause may be seen as a symptom of Alzheimer's disease, rather than the person's rational objection to being taken to the toilet by a stranger.

Stokes suggests that we should see dementia as a barrier to seeing and understanding the person. This strength of the barrier being determined by the person's cognitive and physical status, the disease, compounded by medication and sensory difficulties. According to Stokes:

> When the normal avenues of communication are denied, we cannot readily discover the person. Yet we cannot allow the destruction of understanding who people with dementia are and why they do what they do. If we make contact with the person behind the barrier we are offered the opportunity to stand the prevailing opinion of dementia on its head and assert that much behaviour in dementia is not meaningless, but meaningful. (Stokes 2001, p.55)

In his enhanced model, Stokes stresses the importance of seeing BC within a wider context in which both the social environment (care practices, relationships) and structured environment (architecture, design) are influential.

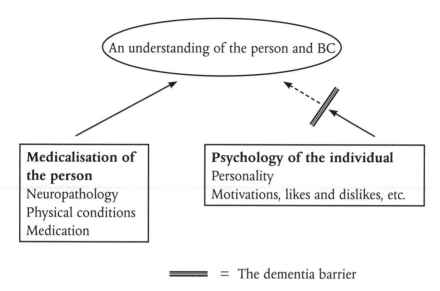

Figure 5.2 The person behind the barrier of the disease (adapted from Stokes 2001)

Kunik's model of behavioural problems (Kunik et al. 2003)

Kunik *et al.* describe their model as a multi-dimensional model of problematic behaviours. They suggest that there are three aspects that one must examine when accounting for such behaviours, namely features associated with the person, the caregiver, and the environment. Each of these aspects is then divided further into fixed and mutable determinants. Fixed determinants are characteristics that are difficult or impossible to change, while mutable characteristics can be altered via the efforts of therapists, family and staff, etc. A truncated version of the model is provided in Figure 5.3.

The model helps to distinguish between 'unchangeable' aspects that provide a context to the BC, and the aspects that can be targeted in any change process. For example, one may not be able to get someone to walk well, but one can assist her to get out of the house on a regular basis by supplying her with a motorised wheel-chair. These regular outings could help with her frustration and reduce the incidences of BC.

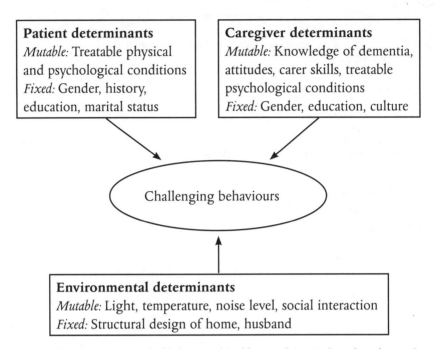

Figure 5.3 Conceptual model of behavioural problems in dementia (Kunik et al. 2003)

Comprehensive model of psychiatric symptoms of progressive degenerative dementia (Volicer and Hurley 2003)

Volicer and Hurley describe their model as integrating behavioural and psychiatric approaches in the understanding and management of BC. Visually, the model is rather reminiscent of a four-ringed sliced onion. At the core is the 'dementia process', which is influenced by the person's premorbid personality and the nature of the dementia. Each of the two inner rings describe the possible primary and secondary causes of the BC. The authors describe these two inner rings as follows:

> Primary consequences of dementia are functional impairment, mood disorders, and delusions and hallucinations. These primary consequences in combination or alone, lead to secondary consequences: inability to initiate meaningful activities, dependence in activities of daily living, spatial disorientation and anxiety. Primary and secondary consequences of dementia cause peripheral symptoms (BC). (Volicer and Hurley 2003)

The outer ring contains the BC (resistiveness, combativeness, food refusal, interference with others, etc.). The model also highlights the role of four contextual factors in influencing the type and severity of the BC displayed; these are caregiving approaches, social environment, physical environment and medical treatment. The authors believe that this model is helpful in treating BC because it forces one to consider the lineage of the problematic behaviours.

Cohen-Mansfield's unmet-needs model (Cohen-Mansfield 2000a)

Cohen-Mansfield's work has already been discussed in Chapters 1 and 2. Her impressive body of work is essential reading for those working in this field. One of her most illuminating models is the 'unmet-needs' perspective (see Figure 5.4), which is similar to the needs-driven behaviour (NDB) model of Algase *et al.* (1996).

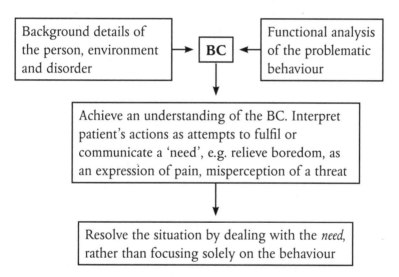

Figure 5.4 Cohen-Mansfield's model of unmet needs (2000a)

The behaviours are viewed as products of an unmet need. The behaviours are therefore: attempts to get the need met; signals relating to one's need; or demonstrations of frustration because a need is not being met. Thus the job of the clinician is to identify the person's need, and this is done by looking at current and historical aspects of the person's life. Once the causal need has been determined the interventions are aimed at meeting the need. Cohen-Mansfield's extension of her unmet needs model was the treatment routes for exploring agitation (TREA) framework (see Chapter 1). It is used in the treatment of different types of agitation (verbal agitation, physical non-aggression and aggressive behaviours) and suggests that these behaviours have different aetiologies and meanings, requiring different treatment strategies. For example, Cohen-Mansfield's (2000a) empirical data suggest that the needs that typically underlie verbal agitation are related to discomfort, lack of social contacts, and physical pain; with inactivity and depression also playing a role (see Figure 5.5). The TREA approach utilises a decision tree to arrive at the most likely cause of the BC based on assessment of the behaviour, the environment and information about the individual's past preferences and needs. The decision tree is used to guide the caregiver to ascertain the need that is most likely to be contributing to the behaviour.

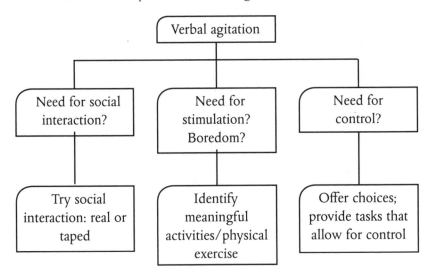

Figure 5.5 Examples of approaches to the management of verbal agitation, from the TREA model

James' challenging behaviour (JCB) conceptualisation (James 2010)

This conceptual model shares many features with Cohen-Mansfield's. It demonstrates that behaviours only tend to be deemed challenging when labelled so by someone else (see Figure 5.6). For example, rummaging through drawers is only challenging when it disturbs another person.

The model suggests that in order to understand a person's need one must determine the person's current view of the world, and how closely that perspective matches the view of her carers (i.e. the norm). In determining whether there is a match, one might want to know: Does the person know where she is? Is she aware of her age? Does she have insight about her strengths and weaknesses? What are her coping strategies? What are her fears? Can she communicate pain? What is bound to annoy her? etc. To understand such things a detailed assessment of her past and present status is required.

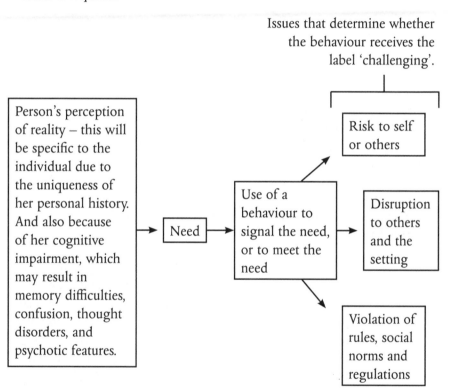

Figure 5.6 James' challenging behaviour (JCB) model

Over a number of years the features of this model have been turned into a clinical framework, which has come to be known as the Newcastle model (see Figure 5.7). This model is discussed in detail in Chapter 6.

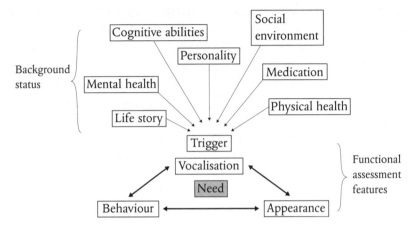

Figure 5.7 Newcastle clinical model (James 1999)

The final section of this chapter illustrates a model commonly used to help carers empathise with the emotions of people with poor communication skills. It is also a useful method for gaining insight into the emotional dynamics of the caring process.

Conceptual model for understanding emotional dynamics
Cognitive triads

BC are associated with a great deal of emotional expression and emotional thinking, both from the person with dementia and the carers. Typically when people are thinking emotionally, they are less rational and more impulsive. During such states their problem-solving abilities are also impaired, and this is clearly not helpful for those with existing cognitive difficulties. Because understanding and recognising emotions are important when one works in a caring role, therapists should spend a lot of time helping carers to detect emotional changes in themselves and in the person with dementia. From Darwin's (1872) theory it is evident that we are good at distinguishing between emotions, and are able to empathise with the states of other people displaying such feelings. Darwin noted that across all cultures of the world humans are able to recognise six basic emotional expressions: anger, depression, anxiety, disgust, surprise, happiness (Ekman 1973). For the present purposes, the themes associated with three key emotions are discussed – depression, anxiety and anger. Beck moved this area further forward with his models of content specificity (Beck 1976). He suggested that people's appearance was linked to certain types of thoughts, which were best illustrated via a cognitive triad (see Table 5.1).

Table 5.1 Cognitive themes and their relationships to emotional appearance

Appearance	Cognitive themes
Depressed	The person has a self-perception of being worthless or inadequate, perceiving the world as hostile or uncaring, and viewing the future as being hopeless.
Anxious	The person has a self-perception of being vulnerable, perceiving her environment to be chaotic, and the future as unpredictable.
Angry	The person perceives that someone is acting unjustly towards her, and her rights are being infringed. Also there is a perception of the environment as being hostile, and a need to act immediately to protect her self-esteem from future harm.

For example, a typical triad for depression would be: 'I'm worthless', 'The world is punishing', 'The future is bleak', whereas the corresponding triad for anxiety would be, 'I'm vulnerable', 'The world is threatening/chaotic,' 'The future is unpredictable'. One can use the cognitive triad format to elucidate the typical thoughts association with the emotion of anger, for example, 'It shouldn't happen to me', 'The world is hostile', 'The future is dangerous' (James 2001).

These triads are particularly useful in the area of BC, especially in situations where one's clients may have poor communication skills. In such circumstances, one is often unable to ask them how they are feeling or what they are thinking. However, by simply looking at their expressions, one can gain some insight to the themes of their distress. Further, the triad is helpful as a treatment template – thus if a therapist sees someone looking anxious, he should simply ask himself (a) What is making Mrs Smith feel vulnerable…is there anything I can do to change this?; (b) Is there anything I can do to make things more predictable?; (c)

What can I do to reduce the chaos within the environment? For example, in Figure 5.8 (below) one can see that Mrs Smith's anger is actually founded on anxiety. Indeed, her anger was because she felt patronised while in a heightened state of arousal, owing to earlier feelings of shame and anxiety. It follows therefore that the treatment should be based on making her feel less panicky, providing her with assistance to find the toilet through better signage and directions, etc.

Anxiety at not being able to locate the toilet
Her expression suggested that she was fearful, and unsure about how she was going to cope in this confusing situation.

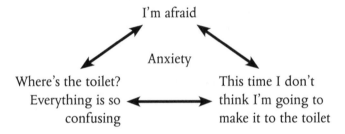

Mrs Smith's fear reduced her ability to think and she got more confused. In her panic she failed to find the toilet in time.

Shame at wetting herself (shame is associated with feelings of humiliation)
Mrs Smith felt humiliated because she had wet herself, and others could see this because of her stained clothes.
Because she felt emotionally charged and did not want to feel shameful anymore, when a carer came to assist and asked her to go to her room and change her trousers, Mrs Smith became aggressive.

Anger because she feels she's been made to look a fool
The triad for anger suggests that Mrs Smith felt she had been treated badly.

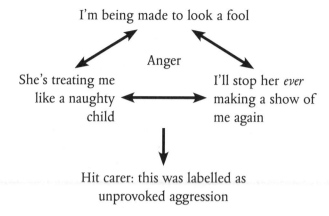

Figure 5.8 Understanding Mrs Smith's anger based on her fear and shame

These triads are also useful when examining the dynamics occurring during BC episodes, providing an opportunity for carers to explore their own reactions to difficult situations. A typical carer example is given below. It highlights the way in which triadic models can be used to support carers to learn to empathise with the experience of their impaired relative through monitoring the care-recipient's mood and behaviour.

Case example

Mrs Taylor (Joan) was a 71-year-old lady attending a group for family carers of people with dementia. Her husband of 52 years (Tom, aged 75) had been diagnosed with Alzheimer's disease three years previously, and had recently started to get up at sun-rise to dress for work as a miner; he was unaware that he was retired. Joan felt helpless and unable to control any aspect of the situation. She was upset that Tom ignored her repeated pleas for him to stop, and was angry that he was refusing to listen to her when she told him he was retired. She also described grieving for the loss of the 'person' that she had known for so many years, and felt guilty for shouting at him.

Following a visit by Joan to her general practitioner, Tom was referred to an older person's community mental health team for assessment of his BC. Once the couple were in contact with health services, Joan was invited to join a carers' group for people with dementia. In common with other group members, Joan was experiencing a number of powerful emotions. She was determined to do the best that she could for her husband, but her physical exhaustion (through lack of sleep) and emotional exhaustion were now getting in the way of her ability to problem-solve day-to-day hassles, thereby increasing her sense of feeling overwhelmed.

Joan obtained benefits from attending the group. Indeed, she felt comforted knowing that she was 'not the only one' to experience feelings of frustration, anger and guilt. However, her increased understanding of her own internal state did not provide any additional insight into her husband's situation. Negative thoughts such as: 'He must know what he's doing' and 'He's never ever listened to me' triggered anger, especially when she had been woken in the morning by him searching for his pit helmet. Yet occasionally as she shouted at him, she could see his discomfort and distress when he seemed to realise that there was some truth in what she was shouting. Typically she'd yell, 'You're an old selfish bastard, you're too weak to walk down the road, never mind work a seam of coal.'

The use of the triadic formulations helped Joan to consider her husband's mental state, and helped her gain insight into the moment-to-moment dynamics of the emotional shifts during their confrontations. Figure 5.9 outlines typical interactions between Mr and Mrs Taylor, starting at the point when Joan found her husband dressing in the morning. Some of the statements attributed to Tom in the triads were generated by Joan and the therapist; and were seen as 'best guesses'. However the 'guesses' are based on observable information about Tom's behaviour, body language and expressed mood rather than assumptions arising from Joan's emotional thinking.

From Figure 5.9, one can see that when Joan sees her husband get up, her anger is triggered and she shouts at him. He is startled and becomes abusive towards her (no-one has shouted at him like this since he was a child!). She responds to his abuse by becoming more aggressive; she is determined that she'll not back down because: 'I can't let him get through the door and be allowed to walk the streets at 5 am.' Tom sometimes becomes aware that something is wrong with his view of things during these arguments. This leads him to become quiet and withdrawn, looking confused and frightened. This response triggers feelings of guilt and depression in Joan.

The process of generating the triadic conceptualisations with the therapist helped Joan to gain a better insight into her husband's perspective, and gave her the opportunity to reappraise the situation. She was able to appreciate that Tom's confused and anxious appearance was inconsistent with her negative thoughts that he was being intentionally stubborn. Thus, Joan was able to reappraise her perspective that he was purposefully 'winding her up', and instead she was able to explore alternative hypotheses for her husband's behaviour. For example, she could begin to see that his behaviour demonstrated that rather than this being a 'different' man, he was still the same conscientious worker he had always been. She even looked proud of him when she stated that he had never been late for work in his life. Also it reminded her of what a good family provider he had been. With help, she was even able to see that his behaviour could be seen as his own attempt to maintain some self-respect, and perhaps he was trying to find security in a role that he had previously done very well.

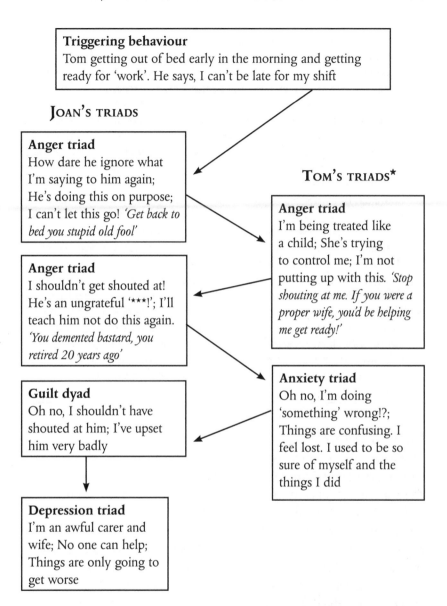

Triggering behaviour
Tom getting out of bed early in the morning and getting ready for 'work'. He says, I can't be late for my shift

JOAN'S TRIADS

Anger triad
How dare he ignore what I'm saying to him again; He's doing this on purpose; I can't let this go! *'Get back to bed you stupid old fool'*

TOM'S TRIADS*

Anger triad
I'm being treated like a child; She's trying to control me; I'm not putting up with this. *'Stop shouting at me. If you were a proper wife, you'd be helping me get ready!'*

Anger triad
I shouldn't get shouted at! He's an ungrateful '***!'; I'll teach him not do this again. *'You demented bastard, you retired 20 years ago'*

Anxiety triad
Oh no, I'm doing 'something' wrong!?; Things are confusing. I feel lost. I used to be so sure of myself and the things I did

Guilt dyad
Oh no, I shouldn't have shouted at him; I've upset him very badly

Depression triad
I'm an awful carer and wife; No one can help; Things are only going to get worse

NB: The quotes in italics is what was actually said, the other material are examples of internal dialogue.

*Owing to Tom's cognitive difficulties, he was unable to provide details of his thoughts about the incidents. Hence, his triads were derived collaboratively between the therapist and Joan. The therapist used specific questions to help her gain better insight and to generate her husband's triad. (e.g. If you were in your husband's position, how might you respond to what was said and how you said it?).

Figure 5.9 Mapping the triads for Mr and Mrs Taylor

Exploration resulted in some practical solutions to reduce the likelihood of the distressing behaviour. For example, putting photographs around the bedroom regarding his work and retirement; mounting the newspaper cutting of the pit closure on the wall next to the bed, and referring to it frequently; removing any 'work-like' clothes (gardening gear, etc.) to another room and leaving only formal dress in the bedroom wardrobe. The hands of the clock were also moved back 2 hours, and when he started to get up Joan would suggest it was still too early for him to be leaving for work. Joan was also shown how to de-escalate the situation by communicating in a calmer manner, because it was evident that shouting at him made him more stubborn. Over time she learned that actually letting him leave the bedroom to potter downstairs by himself often resulted in him re-orientating himself. It was particularly helpful to ask him to bring her up a cup of tea, because by the time he had done this, his intention to go to work had gone. The use of exit alarms was a final precaution to ensure that if he did leave, she would know. Through taking action and seeing changes in Tom's behaviour, Joan's sense of coping increased.

The triadic formulations helped Mrs Taylor to normalise her responses to different situations, understand the dynamics, challenge unhelpful thoughts about herself and generate new interventions. She was able to accept that she was likely to experience the occasional extreme negative emotional response (anger, frustration, transient hate) as a natural part of the caring process. Such acknowledgements served to prevent the exacerbation of guilt and depression, and perhaps the build-up of emotions that may lead on to abuse.

CONCLUSION

Several conceptual models have been presented in this chapter, each covering a slightly different aspect of care and having differing functions. The feature that links them all is that they have attempted to provide an understanding of people's experience of dementia – of the predisposing, triggering, and maintaining factors associated with their distress. Some of the models have also outlined various protective factors that may be enhanced in order to promote well-being (e.g. CoD, James 2010).

As seen on pp.98–104, conceptual models are also useful in understanding the distress of carers. Evidence suggests that by achieving a better understanding of the dynamics associated with BC, carers can reframe the BC in the context of this awareness. Armed with such understanding, carers find it easier to focus on the person rather than on the behaviour (Moniz-Cook, Woods and Gardiner 2000).

Due to these potential benefits, it is hoped the use of conceptualisations will increase in the area of dementia care. Other clinical areas have greatly benefited from their use (Eells et al. 1998), and I feel our speciality could do the same.

Chapter 6

The Newcastle Service: An Illustration of a Specialist Challenging Behaviour Team's Clinical Model

INTRODUCTION

This chapter illustrates how features discussed so far can be applied with a clinical setting. The approach described offers a credible alternative to medication and takes a biopsychosocial view of BC. BC are considered to be as a consequence of an unmet need with the focus of the intervention being to meet the need. By using models that conceptualise the experience of dementia, it is possible to formulate targeted interventions for many of the challenging behaviours exhibited. Thus the following chapter illustrates how the principles and theories outlined above have informed the work of a specialist BC service – the Newcastle Challenging Behaviour Team (NCBT). The service works into 24-hour settings, and provides similar input to other teams in the UK, including the Doncaster Care Homes Liaison Service (Hirst and Oldknow 2009), which is mentioned in national guidelines as an example of good practice.

By the end of the chapter the reader will be aware of the following:

- The key structural and process features of a biopsychosocial framework for treating BC.

- The range of psychotherapeutic skills required to work competently with clients and staff in 24-hour care facilities.

The NCBT approach is called 'Carer-centred, person-focused' due to the fact it is systemic, viewing the staff's responses to the BC as a key factor in both its maintenance and resolution. In relation to the latter, many of the interventions devised are not formal psychological therapies (RO, reminiscence, CST) rather they are bespoke practical strategies (see Tables 2.1–2.6). Indeed, some of the methods may well be techniques previously used by carers, although with limited success due to the lack of consistency in which they were carried out. The rather basic and practical nature of many of the interventions are a crucial feature because within this clinical field, resources are often limited and staff training poor. Therefore, if the treatment strategies are highly sophisticated and require expensive equipment, it is unlikely the approaches will be carried out.

To emphasise the need to work collaboratively with the staff, the LCAPS (listen, clarify, agree, plan, support) principles are presented in Table 6.1. The remainder of this chapter will illustrate the LCAPS principles in action, and how they have underpinned the work of the NCBT.

Table 6.1 LCAPS guidelines for working with care staff

	Principle	Features involved	Adaptations to setting in which behaviour is occurring
Listen	The therapist needs to listen to the various stories relating to the CB from those being affected by the behaviour.	It is important that those affected are allowed to give their views on why the behaviour is happening. This may be the first time they've had the opportunity to give their views, and it is good for them to hear themselves articulating their story; this can produce change in itself. Relevant beliefs and emotions are noted. The therapist's role is to listen and not challenge too much at this stage. Background information is also collected which helps to put the behaviour in context.	*Own home:* Key people to listen to include: the client, the immediate family, GP, and social service staff providing a daily care package. It is important to recognise stress within the family's account and assess the impact this is having on the information being given. It is also helpful to assess the capabilities of the main carers to cope with the situation, and the available resources at their disposal. *Care home:* Speak to the resident, care staff (manager, qualified and unqualified), family and other visitors. The GP and/or psychiatrist may also have a perspective. Useful information is available from the case notes and drug charts. *Inpatient:* Speak to the patient, nurses (qualified, unqualified), psychiatrist and other members of the ward team. It is important to speak to the family members and regular visitors. The ward rounds are an important source of information and communication.

Table 6.1 LCAPS guidelines for working with care staff cont.

	Principle	Features involved	Adaptations to setting in which behaviour is occurring
Clarify	The stories provided need to be checked out and clarified because they often contain contradictory information. The facts of the situation need to be clarified (e.g. What is the behaviour, when it occurs, when not occurring, who is present, etc.)	The therapist armed with the background information, and his knowledge of both dementia and CBs starts to check out some of the inconsistencies in the various stories. His role is also to start imparting relevant information, and to distinguish the facts of the situation from any 'unsupported' assumptions. Another task is to discriminate between the emotionally-based thinking from the factually-based evidence.	Each person providing a perspective is asked questions in order to clarify the emerging story. A gentle questioning style is employed, with direct challenges being avoided where possible. *Own home:* The family's story will be reviewed, and further contextual and historical information obtained. Often the family will be asked to monitor the behaviour in more detail via the use of charts, etc. *Care home:* As above, with additional information obtained from staff and case notes. *Inpatient:* As above, with additional information obtained from other professionals in the inpatient team.
Agree	The therapist must achieve an agreed, unifying version of story that provides possible solutions.	Having assessed the situation, the next step is to produce a single version (story) regarding the behaviour. This normally involves organising a meeting with all those involved in order to get a mutually acceptable version of events.	*Own home:* Specific meeting set-up with family members and people involved in providing care. *Care home:* Specific meeting set-up at the care home with staff; this meeting is known as the Information Sharing Session. As many of staff as possible are asked to attend (see detailed description in this chapter). *Inpatient:* The story is developed during the ward rounds and conveyed to other staff at 'daily handovers'.

Plan	Therapist must develop a treatment strategy collaboratively with the person and carers to deal with the problematic situation.	The mutually agreed story provides the platform from which treatment strategies are developed. These strategies also need to be agreed in the presence of everyone in order that the treatment rationale and aims can be clarified and agreed respectively.	*Own home:* Family often require a lot of structure and guidance in developing a workable plan. *Care home:* A care plan is required; one that provides clear and concise information. It is important that the plan is devised with the aid of staff in order that they perceive they have ownership of the care plan. *Inpatient:* As above.
Support	The therapist should support the implementation of the treatment strategy.	If a new treatment approach has been devised, it will often require guidance, modelling, etc. to facilitate implementation. In some circumstances no particular strategy is deemed appropriate, and thus people may require support to enable them to tolerate the ongoing behaviour better.	*Own home:* This may take the form of written instructions, modelling, telephone support. *Care home:* As above, details of the plan may be shared with the care home inspectors. *Inpatient:* As above. However, the greater knowledge base and experience of the staff means that one must be careful not to come across as patronising.

PROTOCOL OF THE NEWCASTLE APPROACH

There are a number of stages to consider when using the NCBT's 14 week (5 + 9 week programme) approach and these are outlined in Table 6.2. As one can see, it is a 'front loaded' method of working, with most of the intensive work taking place in the first 5 weeks of the case. In the later stages the therapist tends to be monitoring and tweaking both the formulation and interventions as a consequence of staff feedback.

Table 6.2 The stages of the '5 plus 9' NCBT treatment model

Guiding ethos: When using the approach in care settings, it is always important for staff to feel they are involved in the various stages of the work; from the assessment to the delivery of the intervention.
Weeks 1–5: Intensive treatment phase
Week 1: Having received the referral, and been allocated the case, the therapist commences the 'fact finding' process. An important step is to make sure that all the physical checks have been completed by the medical practitioner to ensure that the problematic behaviour has not arisen from either an acute infection or transient difficulty (e.g. pain resulting from a fall, constipation). A review of the medication used is also undertaken, and rationalised as appropriate.
Week 2: By the second week, the therapist will have made contact with the home on a number of occasions and spoken to the relevant people, including the client. In conversation with staff, it is made clear what the NCBT's expectations are. To reinforce this, an information sheet is left with the home describing the team's and staff's responsibilities in delivering the package of care. During this week further information is collected from the various sources, and a detailed analysis of the behaviour is undertaken via monitoring charts. The main goal at this stage is to listen to people's accounts of the BC in order to obtain a full account. Unless there are issues to do with safety or risk, it would not be common to challenge staff practices at this point, as this may interfere with relationships with carers. A pre-treatment measure is undertaken with the client's key worker (i.e. neuropsychiatric inventory, Cummings *et al.* 1994).
Week 3: The information collected thus far starts to undergo analysis, and greater clarification of the problems are made. If not done previously, the feedback from the family is added to the growing data set.

Week 4/5: The main event taking place in this phase is the delivery of the information sharing session (ISS). This is a specific session, attended by staff in the care setting (ideally with all levels of staff represented), lasting approximately an hour. In these sessions, the information about the person's problematic behaviour is presented in the context of his/her background. The idea of the session is to develop an understanding of the behaviour in relation to the wider context, allowing staff to speculate on the client's needs, namely, what is driving the behaviour. In terms of the LCAPS model, this phase involves developing the agreed, unifying story with respect to the BC. This process helps to inform the interventions, which are developed and planned by staff during the ISS. One of the goals of the NCBT therapist is to ensure that the planned interventions devised meet the specific measurable achievable relevant and timely (SMART) criteria.

The therapist facilitates the meeting using effective questioning techniques, feedback, summarising, education, challenging strategies, and guided reflection techniques. These methods are designed to get the staff to 'step back' from the situation, and look afresh at the behaviour within its historical and situational context. Collaboration with staff is particularly important when trying to identify the client's needs and possible interpretation of the situation.

Thus the goal of the ISS is to assist staff to become more knowledgeable, empowered and motivated to improve the client's well-being, through the setting of appropriate interventions. Within the process, an effective ISS will have used information from many sources to give staff an understanding of what factors are contributing towards the client's actions. Within this approach, it is vital that the interventions are developed by the staff, so that they have ownership of the treatment process.

Week 6 onwards: Tweaking and support phase

Week 6: Following the ISS, it is the therapist's responsibility to take away the details discussed at the meeting, and recorded on the flip chart, to produce an A4 summary sheet (aka formulation, Figure 6.1). Attached to the formulation sheet will be a detailed description of the interventions (i.e. a care plan, Sells and Shirley 2010). A vital feature underpinning the success of the interventions is that they are carried out consistently and uniformly by all staff. To gauge how well the information is disseminated, the home is provided with a sheet which all staff must sign to indicate that they have read and understood the care plan.

**Table 6.2 The stages of the '5 plus 9'
NCBT treatment model *cont.***

Weeks 7–11: The remaining sessions involve the support of staff, visiting the home to ensure the interventions are being carried out consistently. In some cases, the formulation may require changing or the interventions tweaking.

Weeks 12–14: Unless there are exceptional reasons for continuing input, this milestone results in discharge. At this meeting a discharge interview takes place, where the key worker is asked to complete a qualitative and quantitative (NPI) measure of change.

In the following sub-sections the process and structural features of the approach are described from assessment through to outcome: Process and structural features of the Assessment phase (next section); Information sharing session (p.117); Formulation (p.117); Treatment planning and support (p.122); Assessing the impact of the service (p.122).

PROCESS AND STRUCTURAL FEATURES OF THE ASSESSMENT PHASE: LISTENING AND GENTLY CLARIFYING

The function of the assessment is twofold: first to collect relevant data to help inform the intervention; and second to collect the information in a manner that increases the involvement of staff. In order to achieve these aims the therapist must spend a lot of time listening carefully to various accounts of the BC (see LCAPS), and the strategies used by the carers to deal with them. Unless the current practices require immediate attention, the carers' accounts should not be challenged directly until a good appreciation of the situation is achieved. As the story of the BC begins to emerge some clarification is always necessary, but again this is usually done in a gentle non-confrontational manner. The latter requires therapeutic engagement with the staff: empathising; collaborating; asking exploratory questions (see Table 6.3, adapted from Fossey and James 2007). Indeed, it is by using such processes that the NCBT therapist can encourage staff to become inquisitive and want to learn more about the client and the causes of the BC.

Table 6.3 Some of the skills required to work with staff in care facilities

Technique	Definition	Examples: statements you might hear NCBT member say with respect to theme
Setting goals regarding discussions about client	Negotiating with the staff about the contents and preferred methods of discussing the client's behaviour.	Today we're going to be discussing Ellen's behaviour and some of the reasons for her communicating this way. In your view what are the three things it's essential that we talk through before finishing the session?
Collaborating	Ensuring the staff feel part of the teaching process, encouraging them to be active participants.	You've had lots of experience of this, so before I discuss this issue further, who can tell us what's the best thing to say to her when she calls you a 'bitch'.
Gathering information	Fact finding and obtaining information from the staff about the situation, feelings, thoughts and/or behaviours.	What time does she tend to wake up? What expression did she have on her face after she hit you?
Feedback	Providing specific feedback that aids learning, and asking for feedback to help guide the teaching.	The previous care plan was too vague. The ideas we have discussed today are much clearer and specific, well done!
Summarising/ clarifying	Chunking information to help clarify links and highlight key features.	Great, now let's see if I understand what you did there. You saw her searching for the toilet, and knew she'd be too embarrassed to ask you, so you asked if she'd like to wash her hands and then guided her to the sink in the toilet.

Table 6.3 Some of the skills required to work with staff in care facilities *cont.*

Technique	Definition	Examples: statements you might hear NCBT member say with respect to theme
Supporting and understanding	Providing verbal and non-verbal signs that provide reassurance and encouragement to the staff.	That was difficult, but you seemed to have handled it really, really well.
Informing/ educating	Providing factual information aimed at increasing staff's knowledge.	Multi-infarct dementia is a type of vascular dementia. It is often very difficult to distinguish multi-infarct from Alzheimer's disease.
Aiding reflection	Working with the staff to get them to think through issues in order to come to an increased understanding of key issues.	Let's stop a second and think through the implications of this. If, indeed, pain is a common cause of challenging behaviour, what should we do?
Formulating	Working with the staff to develop a framework that helps to explain residents' behaviours and needs.	OK, we seem to have gathered quite a lot of information about Ellen now. Let's put it all together and see how it helps explain why she's so depressed.
Self-disclosing	Informing staff about personal experiences that help to illustrate issues or concepts.	I must admit, I wasn't aware that diabetes was a side-effect of anti-psychotic use. One of the nurses told me during our training session two weeks ago.
Challenging	Getting the staff to rethink their views, often by pointing out inconsistencies in their thinking.	Well, both of you can't be right. One of you is saying she is like this with everyone, while the other thinks she is cooperative when with certain individuals.

| Disagreeing | Taking a different viewpoint to the staff, in order to highlight an alternative perspective. | I am going have to disagree with that. She is not just being awkward. Remember she has a dementia and thus can struggle at times to make sense of what is happening to her during personal care tasks. |
| Behavioural tasks | Using activity based tasks (role-play, modelling) to help demonstrate skills. | Now that we have discussed the problems and possible strategies for communicating with Ellen, let's try to demonstrate it via a role play. |

It is evident from Table 6.3 that good interpersonal skills are required to work in a care setting. Further it is my belief that the skills of a competent clinician in this area would match the abilities of a therapist working in any other area of mental health.

One of the skills listed in Table 6.3 is formulating. A formulation is the structural framework which summarises the story of the BC. The contents of this framework are outlined in detail on pp.117–121 and presented diagrammatically in Figure 6.1. Completed examples of these formulations are presented in Chapter 7. Copies of these formulations are produced on A4 sheets for every person seen by the NCBT.

The background information (personal histories, health status, etc.) used to inform the formulation is collected from family and staff. These features were discussed in detail in Chapter 2. Diaries and assessment charts are also used to identify the triggers, and further details about the BC. An example of one of the assessment charts used by the service was presented in Chapter 2, Figures 2.1 and 2.2.

The NCBT routinely uses the Neuropsychiatric Inventory (Cummings, Mega, Gray *et al.* 1994) as a pre/post assessment measure; the version used includes the caregiver distress scale (i.e. the NPI-D, see Chapter 2). Details about the impact of the service are discussed later (p.122).

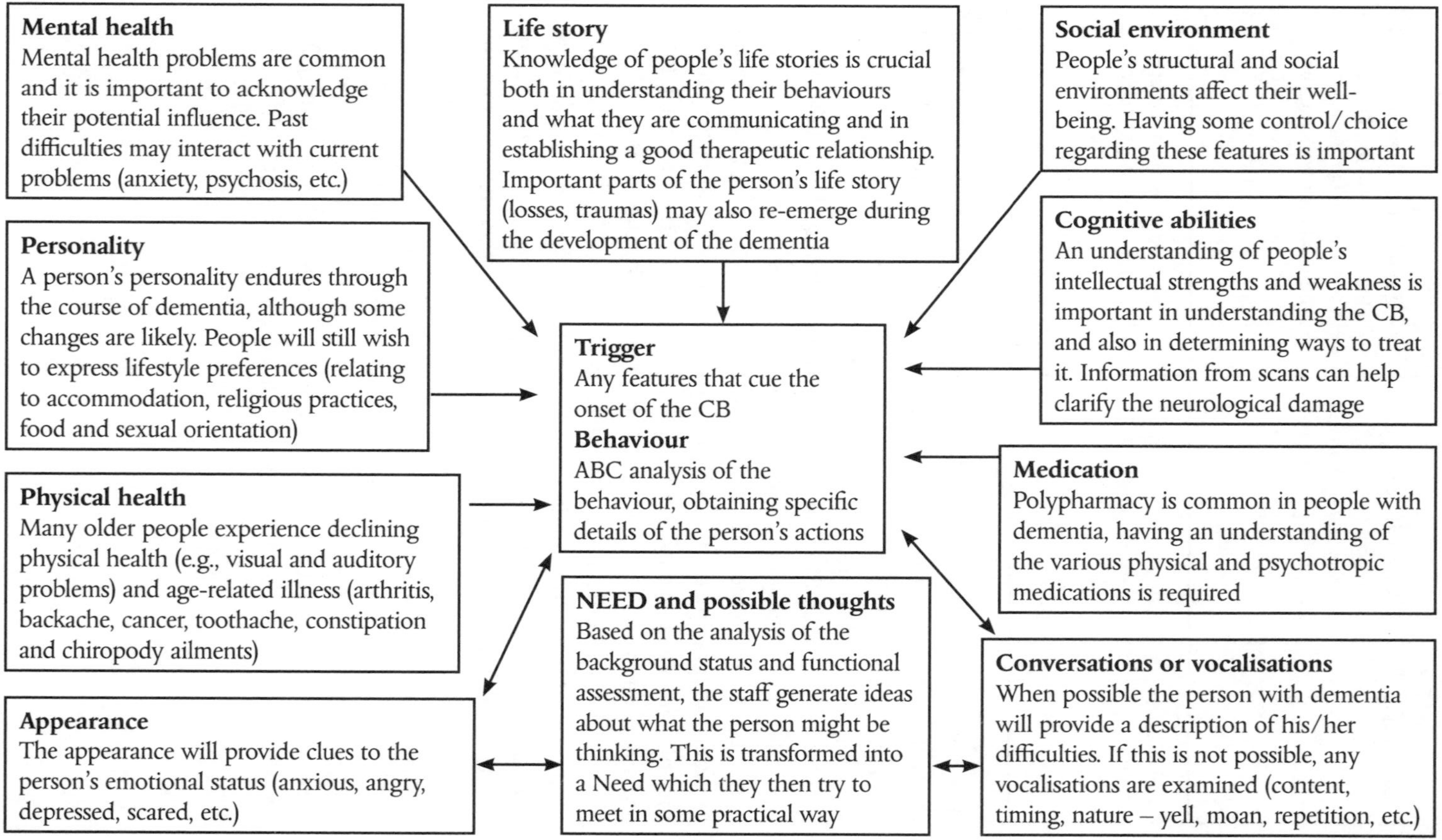

Social environment
People's structural and social environments affect their well-being. Having some control/choice regarding these features is important

Cognitive abilities
An understanding of people's intellectual strengths and weakness is important in understanding the CB, and also in determining ways to treat it. Information from scans can help clarify the neurological damage

Medication
Polypharmacy is common in people with dementia, having an understanding of the various physical and psychotropic medications is required

Conversations or vocalisations
When possible the person with dementia will provide a description of his/her difficulties. If this is not possible, any vocalisations are examined (content, timing, nature – yell, moan, repetition, etc.)

Life story
Knowledge of people's life stories is crucial both in understanding their behaviours and what they are communicating and in establishing a good therapeutic relationship. Important parts of the person's life story (losses, traumas) may also re-emerge during the development of the dementia

Trigger
Any features that cue the onset of the CB

Behaviour
ABC analysis of the behaviour, obtaining specific details of the person's actions

NEED and possible thoughts
Based on the analysis of the background status and functional assessment, the staff generate ideas about what the person might be thinking. This is transformed into a Need which they then try to meet in some practical way

Mental health
Mental health problems are common and it is important to acknowledge their potential influence. Past difficulties may interact with current problems (anxiety, psychosis, etc.)

Personality
A person's personality endures through the course of dementia, although some changes are likely. People will still wish to express lifestyle preferences (relating to accommodation, religious practices, food and sexual orientation)

Physical health
Many older people experience declining physical health (e.g. visual and auditory problems) and age-related illness (arthritis, backache, cancer, toothache, constipation and chiropody ailments)

Appearance
The appearance will provide clues to the person's emotional status (anxious, angry, depressed, scared, etc)

Figure 6.1 Overview of the NCBT's formulation

INFORMATION SHARING SESSION (ISS): OBTAINING AGREEMENT

As seen in Table 6.2, the ISS occurs around week 5. In the ISS, all the background information collected is presented and put together with the data from the behavioural charts. Patterns are explored and detected, potential triggers elucidated, staff are encouraged to relate their experiences of the behaviour and then issues are clarified regarding these accounts. A major part of this work is done via careful questioning skills that help identify patterns and generate hypotheses. For example, if a BC is believed to be associated with pain, then questioning should reveal a pain-related pattern (tooth pain – problems throughout the day, perhaps more frequent when the person is eating or drinking; arthritic pain – worse in morning, or when person is moving or being moved). If the hypothesis is to do with overstimulation, then the BC should be more common during busy times of the day, or when the telephone rings, or when lots of things are happening at the same time. It is my belief that the art of good questioning skills should not be under-estimated, because many hypotheses can be supported or dismissed on the basis of one or two effective questions (James, Morse and Howarth 2010).

The goal of the ISS is to arrive at a single unifying account of the problem (i.e. the story) and develop a plan to deal with it. The plans may include revisions of previous carer strategies that were partially successful. However, in the revised context they may require some modification or to be used more consistently. In terms of the Newcastle model, the problematic behaviour is perceived as an expression of an unmet need on the part of the resident (Cohen-Mansfield 2000a). By the end of the ISS a set of interventions and approaches will have been developed in collaboration with the staff. It is relevant to note that the therapist plays a major role in ensuring that the goals are realistic and feasible. Indeed, for each intervention that therapist is routinely instructed to employ the SMART (specific, measurable, achievable, relevant, timely) criteria with respect to the goal setting (Fossey and James 2007). Further discussion about the goals is presented in the section on Treatment Planning and Support (p.122).

FORMULATION: UNIFYING STORY

Following the information sharing session (ISS), a formulation is produced (see Figure 6.1 and case examples in Chapter 7). Much of the information in Figure 6.1 will already have been presented to the staff in the ISS via a flip chart. This flip chart information will have helped generate discussion and assisted the staff to achieve a greater level of understanding regarding the resident's behaviour. However, with respect to the formulation, the information is condensed and written-up in the form of a single A-4 sheet of paper. The experience of the Newcastle team suggests that supplying staff with an overly comprehensive formulation presented on multiple sheets is both offputting and less likely to be read. In contrast, it has been found that a single formulation sheet with a brief care plan attached provides the most effective treatment strategy.

The components presented in Figure 6.1 are in two parts: (i) The background features (physical health, personality, mental health, life story, social environment, cognitive abilities, medication); and (ii) The functional assessment of the BC (triggers, behaviour, vocalisations, appearance).

Background features

A description of the background features has been provided in Chapter 2, and presented diagrammatically in the Iceberg model, Figure 1.1. It is relevant to note that information on all the background factors is obtained by examining case files, speaking to carers and relatives, and the person with dementia where possible. Specific forms have been devised by the NCBT to aid data collection, such as the personal profile questionnaires. These are questionnaires given to the family that ask about the person's past, likes, dislikes, coping style, favourite pastimes, foods, music preferences, etc.

Functional assessment of the BC

Figure 6.1 shows a triangle comprised of three themes: vocalisation, appearance and behaviour. The framework uses this triad to understand the client's thinking and experiences of the episode of BC. One way of finding out what a person is experiencing is to talk to her. However, the person with dementia may not always be able to tell you what is driving her behaviour. Valuable information can be gained simply by observing the person. There are three key features to pay attention to:

- the person's behaviour
- what they say and/or vocalise (whether coherent or not)
- how they appear to be feeling (i.e. the person's appearance and facial expression).

These observations can give us important clues to clients' beliefs and what they are thinking; such information helps towards a better understanding of their needs. It is relevant to note that if there is more than one challenging behaviour present, there will be more than one trigger and triad.

Triggers

The box labelled 'triggers' is situated between the background details and the triad. This box simply highlights the circumstances in which the problematic behaviours are observed.

Behaviour

Part of the assessment involves gathering details of what exactly happens during an episode of BC (i.e. a functional assessment). General labels such as 'aggression' or 'wandering' tell us little about what a person is actually doing, and less about why they are doing it. Thus a careful analysis of the behaviour is essential.

Such an analysis will need to consider antecedents and consequences, and where and with whom the behaviour does and does not occur (see Figure 6.1).

Conversations or vocalisations

It is helpful to gather information about the clients' difficulties by asking them directly. Most of this information will come from conversations and listening to the person. The verbal communications of people with severe dementia are not always coherent. However, it is important to take into account the type of vocalisation (shouting, type of screaming – pain related, calling for help), when it occurs and its content (the words used).

Appearance

It is important to observe the client's appearance. Do they look anxious, depressed or angry? Observing how the person appears is key to understanding their experiences. The three most common forms of emotional distress are anxiety, anger and depression. Empirical research informs us that each of these has a characteristic theme associated with it (Beck 1976; James 2001). These themes are outlined in Table 6.4.

Table 6.4 Cognitive themes and their relationships to emotional appearance

Appearance	Cognitive themes
Depressed	The person has a self-perception of being worthless or inadequate, perceiving the world as hostile or uncaring, and viewing the future as being hopeless.
Anxious	The person has a self-perception of being vulnerable, perceiving her environment to be chaotic, and the future as unpredictable.
Angry	The person perceives that someone is acting unjustly towards her, and her rights are being infringed. Also there is a perception of the environment as being hostile, and a need to act immediately to protect her self-esteem from future harm.

As described above, when someone is feeling anxious, they often see themselves as vulnerable and unable to cope with the demands of the situation. When someone appears depressed, they often see themselves as inadequate, worthless and the situation as being hopeless. Finally, when someone is angry, they tend to see themselves as having been badly treated or misused in some way. Understanding these signs helps to inform us what people's needs might be. The anxious person may be fearful for his safety, needing to be helped to feel less vulnerable. The depressed person will need to be given a greater sense of worth, while the angry resident will need to feel her rights are not being infringed.

Need and possible thoughts

The behaviour, vocalisation and appearance observed during an episode of BC, when combined with the background information, can be used to try to understand what is causing the problem. Part of our role is to try to get staff to empathise with the person's situation, to think what his beliefs are and what he might be thinking in that situation and to try to understand the reasons behind the BC. In other words, the aim is for staff to develop a 'theory of mind' perspective with respect to the person with dementia. Table 6.5 summarises how the information obtained above can be used in devising appropriate interventions.

Table 6.5 Illustration of how the emotional presentation of the person can help identify need and develop the intervention

Emotional appearance	Themes	BC associated with the theme	Need	Possible actions to deal with theme
Angry when carer removes her dinner plate without asking whether the client has finished	She thinks she is not being shown enough respect	Swearing at staff: Your filthy bitches	To be respected	Prior to touching her plate, ask the client whether she enjoyed the meal and then whether she's finished
Depressed and lonely when sees other resident has a visitor	Thinks no one wants her	Sits by herself, refusing to eat	To feel valued by others	At visiting times assign a member of staff to spend some 1:1 time with her
Shame followed by *Anger* when member of staff points out to the client that she has been incontinent	Initial theme is to do with a sense of embarrassment, but due to her reduced range of coping strategies to deal with the situation, she goes on the offensive	Threw cup of water on floor and told staff member to f*ck off. Swore again when staff tried to change her.	To have her dignity maintained, while requiring to assist her change her wet clothes (hygiene/ skin integrity reasons)	Use of a therapeutic lie (James *et al.* 2006d), informing her that she must've spilled some water over herself. Hence would she like some assistance to get changed

TREATMENT PLANNING AND SUPPORT

As stated above, the interventions are based on carers' suggestions and are developed and refined at the end of the information sharing session with the therapist's help. After the group meeting, it is the therapist's role to take away the suggestions and put them together into a coherent treatment plan. As a result a new care plan is produced based around the problematic behaviour. The care plans are honed down to the bare essentials because once again it is found that overly complex treatment goals are not adhered to and often not read.

Over the preceding weeks the carers are supported in their implementation of the plans, and the strategies are tweaked as required in order to meet the needs of the client and also the carer. This support may take the form of advice, modelling and teaching.

In Chapter 7 some of the common treatment strategies that have been employed by the NCBT are presented (see Table 7.3). The key thing to note is the simplicity of many of the interventions. For example, helping the staff to communicate better with the resident, organising regular trips out of the care setting, enabling the person to exercise more choice in her daily routine. Also see the intervention tables described in Chapter 2, Tables 2.1–2.6.

ASSESSING THE IMPACT OF THE SERVICE

This section describes the impact of the NCBT through the results of an audit that examined feedback from work undertaken in care homes (Wood-Mitchell *et al.* 2007b). The audit looked at the outcome data of two specialist nurses and an assistant psychologist in the NCBT between September 2005, and September 2006. The statistical data were taken from the team's outcome measure, the neuropsychiatric inventory (NPI, Cummings, Mega, Gray *et al.* 1994). The NPI is a measure which gives an overall BC score based on the severity and frequency scores of 12 psychiatric symptoms (maximum NPI score = 144). The team use the NPI-D version of the scale, which also measures carer-giver distress (D) (maximum D score = 60).

For each resident, a member of staff in the care home who knew the resident well was asked to complete an NPI-D pre- and post-treatment. All informants were senior carers, or general/mental health nurses who were involved in the care of the resident.

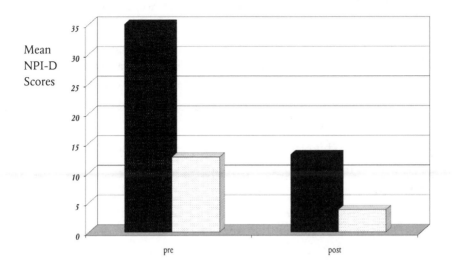

Figure 6.2 NPI results for NCBT outcome audit (Dark=NPT score, Light=Caregiver distress score

The results from the audit are presented in Figure 6.2, and reveal a significant difference in the pre-intervention and post-intervention behavioural scores. The post-intervention behavioural scores (mean 13.61, s.d. 9.51) were significantly lower than the pre-intervention behavioural scores (mean 35.05, s.d. 22.43). There was also a significant difference between the pre-intervention and post-intervention scores for caregiver distress (mean = 11.72, s.d. = 7.60 and mean = 3.77, s.d. = 3.65 respectively). Additionally, during the periods specified above only three residents (6.1%) were admitted to hospital and three were relocated to another care setting. Jointly, these findings suggest that the NCBT's approach is an effective method for reducing BC and staff distress.

In terms of transfers and hospital admissions, although one cannot be certain of the numbers of residents who would have been relocated, it is likely that a number of these complex cases would have been admitted due to their high initial NPI-D scores. Qualitative analysis of the impact of the team has also been undertaken with the key-workers of residents who had been treated successfully by the team (Scott 2009). As part of this survey, the key-workers were asked to comment on what they found helpful about the input of the NCBT. Here are a number of the comments:

- 'We are now more tolerant, now that we know about her background.'

- 'We have more understanding...we now recognise what we thought was verbal aggression was just her way of bantering with us – she's very sarcastic, but that's her nature' (manager).

- 'Staff's understanding has increased... staff understand why she is unable to inhibit these behaviours.'

- 'Talking to him... Staff reading the handouts made them change their approaches towards him.'

- 'We have more information on her so we can talk to her.'

- 'She does still have "bad days" but we recognise it tends to happen when certain staff are on duty – staff who do not adhere to the plan.'

CONCLUSION

This chapter has provided a detailed account of how the NCBT operates. It demonstrates how the various models and frameworks described in the earlier chapters are used clinically. Every person referred to the service is offered this comprehensive approach, although sometimes the full 14-week course may not be required. As one can see, while the work is designed to increase the well-being of the person with dementia, the changes require the involvement of the carers. Hence getting the carers on board is a key element in our 'carer-centred, person-focused' therapy. The final section of the chapter provided data regarding the success of the approach, and included some favourable comments from staff who had worked with the NCBT.

It is worth noting that the above approach has been criticised for being time-consuming and too resource intensive. In its defence, it is important to note the high degree of complexity of many of the conditions treated, particularly the chronic ones. Further, in relation to younger clients, we would regard a 14-week programme as a short-term therapy. Indeed, in adult services those prescribed psychodynamic therapy may receive 1 to 2 years of intensive treatment.

Chapter 7

Case Studies

INTRODUCTION

Four case examples are described, each illustrating some of the theories and frameworks discussed in the previous chapters. The case material is taken from the work of the Newcastle Challenging Behaviour Team (NCBT). Other information for this chapter has been obtained from various audits of the NCBT conducted by trainee Clinical Psychologists at Newcastle University, UK (Cunningham 2005; Makin 2009; Scott 2009).

By the end of the chapter the reader will be aware of the following:

- How to use biopsychosocial models in the treatment of common BC.

- The manner in which formulations directly inform people's care plans.

- The interventions in the care plans are extremely practical, requiring few resources and little/no training. This is because the carers in the settings tend to have limited resources and training.

The cases have been chosen to illustrate the breadth of presentations seen by the team. The first case, Gordon, is the most typical example as he presented with aggression, particularly when receiving help with personal-care. John, case two, was treated for sexual disinhibition. This is a type of behaviour that many carers find difficult to deal with, and can lead to multiple transfers of the person within the care sector. The third case presents Isabel, whose care was transformed once her daughter was able to provide details of her mother's long-standing personality issues. Further investigation, and use of a carer questionnaire, resulted in a diagnosis of Asperger's syndrome that helped inform Isabel's care plan. The final case example presents Betsy who was treated in her own home. This treatment was undertaken with the assistance of her husband and with the support of the rest of her family.

In the final section of the chapter, a summary of the interventions typically used by the NCBT is presented.

Case examples

Case 1: Gordon

Reason for referral

Gordon, aged 67, suffered from moderately severe Alzheimer's disease. At the time of referral he had been in a elderly mentally infirm (EMI) nursing category care home for 2 years. He was presenting with restlessness, going into other residents' rooms and putting on their clothes. He was refusing to leave his room and was physically aggressive towards staff, particularly during personal care interventions. He also followed staff around, which some staff perceived as threatening, describing it as 'stalking'.

Assessment

The assessment involved listening to Gordon, his care staff and family members. A helpful interview was also undertaken with the home's manager and a qualified nurse about the current shift patterns which seemed to impact on his behaviour. It became apparent from the discussions that the staff had developed a negative attitude towards him, and were hoping he would be transferred to another home. This view was supported by the GP, following an incident in which Gordon hit him.

Many staff thought that his behaviour was 'attention seeking', claiming that he was aware of how much his actions annoyed others. Prior to the information sharing session (ISS), details were gathered about Gordon's background. ABC charts were used to better describe the episodes of challenging behaviour. These details helped to develop some hypotheses about the causes of the BC, and generated some queries requiring further clarification. Examples of some of the therapist's queries are presented in Table 7.1. It is relevant to note that openly seeking clarification is a very powerful process as it gently challenges inconsistencies and gets the staff to reflect further on the facts and to generate new ideas.

**Table 7.1 Queries and responses: demonstrating
how therapists' questions can help illuminate
features underpinning the BC**

Query from therapist	Carer response – clues about the nature of the behaviour can be found in the reply
When walking around the home, how does Gordon appear – angry, threatening, confused or anxious?	It depends. If you stop him and try to take him into a room, he gets angry. He likes to do things for himself; he'll only do what he wants. Mind you he's very nosey, and notices whenever we've made changes. After we moved furniture or something, he'll come and check things out.
Does Gordon get angry every time you try to take him to the toilet? Do you think Jim does anything differently with him?	Almost every time. He's a bit better with Jim, but even Jim struggles in the evenings. Jim is chilled. May be a bit too chilled for the new home manager. Jim just lets Gordon get on with things. He doesn't mind if Gordon misses the toilet, he's happy to clear it up.
You say that Gordon 'trails' you. When he is walking close to you, does he have a menacing expression on his face?	No, no…he doesn't really have any expression. He look blank, perhaps a bit lost. He sometimes asks for his wife when you ask him what he's doing.

The value of the questions were that they demonstrated the inherent complexity of Gordon's behaviours. Further, the responses showed that labels such as 'wandering' or 'trailing' were misleading descriptions of what was happening. The staff's responses to the queries were also helpful in providing ideas that were later 'worked-up' into interventions. Many of the questions were asked within the ISS. By the end of the ISS, sufficient information was obtained to devise the formulation (see Figure 7.1). The staff had also been helped to produce hypothesis-driven interventions which were then written-up as care plans. The care plans were enclosed with the A4 formulation sheet and given to the care home and family.

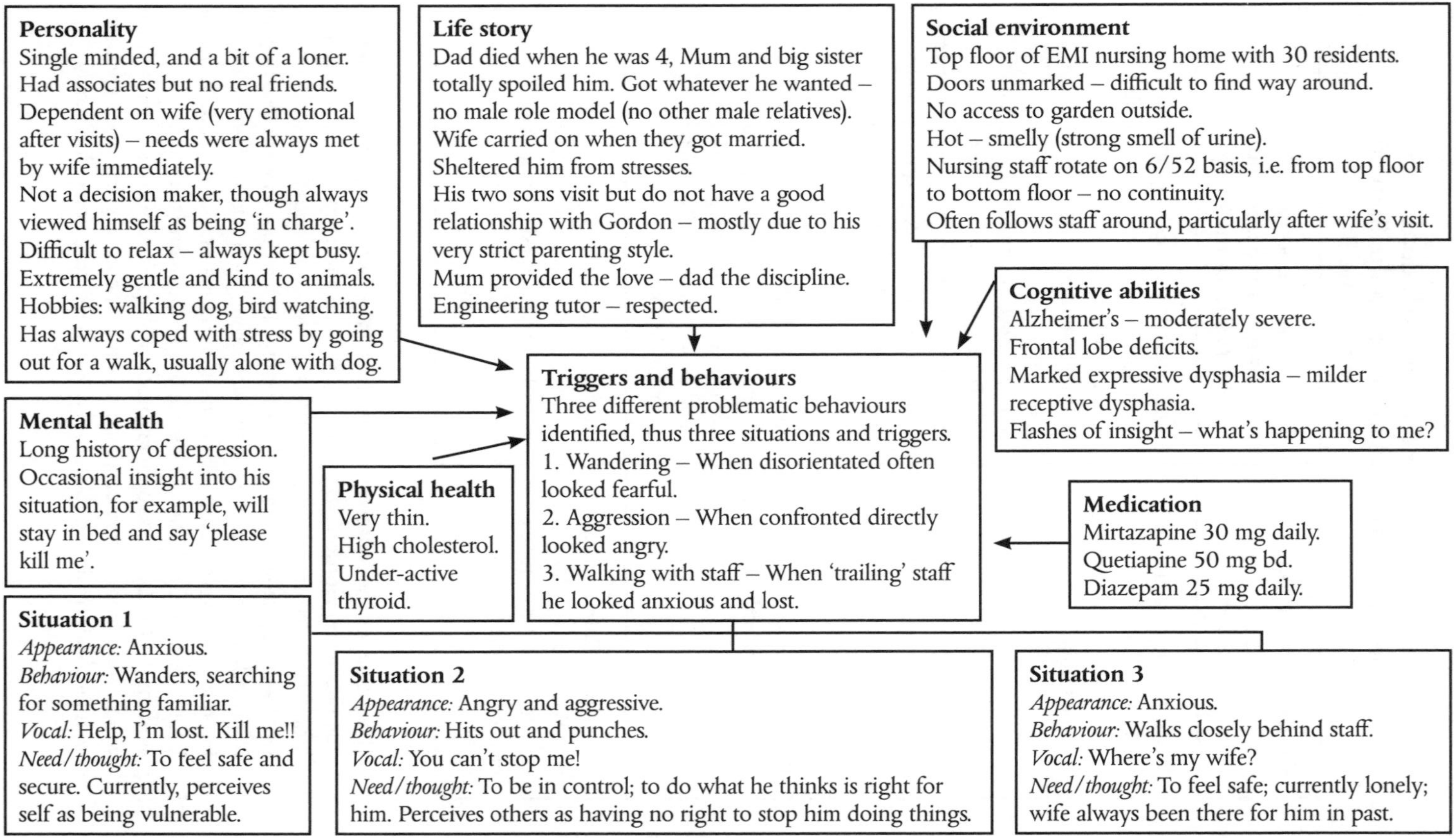

Personality

Single minded, and a bit of a loner.
Had associates but no real friends.
Dependent on wife (very emotional after visits) – needs were always met by wife immediately.
Not a decision maker, though always viewed himself as being 'in charge'.
Difficult to relax – always kept busy.
Extremely gentle and kind to animals.
Hobbies: walking dog, bird watching.
Has always coped with stress by going out for a walk, usually alone with dog.

Life story

Dad died when he was 4, Mum and big sister totally spoiled him. Got whatever he wanted – no male role model (no other male relatives).
Wife carried on when they got married.
Sheltered him from stresses.
His two sons visit but do not have a good relationship with Gordon – mostly due to his very strict parenting style.
Mum provided the love – dad the discipline.
Engineering tutor – respected.

Social environment

Top floor of EMI nursing home with 30 residents.
Doors unmarked – difficult to find way around.
No access to garden outside.
Hot – smells (strong smell of urine).
Nursing staff rotate on 6/52 basis, i.e. from top floor to bottom floor – no continuity.
Often follows staff around, particularly after wife's visit.

Cognitive abilities

Alzheimer's – moderately severe.
Frontal lobe deficits.
Marked expressive dysphasia – milder receptive dysphasia.
Flashes of insight – what's happening to me?

Medication

Mirtazapine 30 mg daily.
Quetiapine 50 mg bd.
Diazepam 25 mg daily.

Mental health

Long history of depression.
Occasional insight into his situation, for example, will stay in bed and say 'please kill me'.

Physical health

Very thin.
High cholesterol.
Under-active thyroid.

Triggers and behaviours

Three different problematic behaviours identified, thus three situations and triggers.

1. Wandering – When disorientated often looked fearful.
2. Aggression – When confronted directly looked angry.
3. Walking with staff – When 'trailing' staff he looked anxious and lost.

Situation 1

Appearance: Anxious.
Behaviour: Wanders, searching for something familiar.
Vocal: Help, I'm lost. Kill me!!
Need/thought: To feel safe and secure. Currently, perceives self as being vulnerable.

Situation 2

Appearance: Angry and aggressive.
Behaviour: Hits out and punches.
Vocal: You can't stop me!
Need/thought: To be in control; to do what he thinks is right for him. Perceives others as having no right to stop him doing things.

Situation 3

Appearance: Anxious.
Behaviour: Walks closely behind staff.
Vocal: Where's my wife?
Need/thought: To feel safe; currently lonely; wife always been there for him in past.

Figure 7.1 Gordon's formulation sheet

Interventions

The Newcastle framework is a biopsychosocial perspective, so in addition to the psychological interventions, changes were made to the medication and to the organisation. Hence, the first step involved a medication review, which revealed that the diazepam was having a paradoxical impact. Thus instead of having a sedative effect, it was making him more agitated. In relation to the organisational change, it was apparent that Gordon struggled when being nursed by people he perceived as unfamiliar. This was exacerbated in this home owing to a full rotation of staff every 6 weeks. From the comments made by staff, Gordon was always more unsettled just after a rotation. On reflection, the manager recognised that the 'lack of continuity' was a problem for a number of the residents, and not just for Gordon. Therefore the shift system was changed, resulting in shorter and more frequent rotations.

The following instructions formed part of the Care Plan, and are based on the staff's own ideas about how to improve their interactions with him.

Instructions recorded in the Care Plan

1. Preventing triggers of Gordon's BC.

   ° Reduce his confusion and help him to remain as independent as possible. He needs to feel he has some control. For example, let him have his meals in his room when he requests. Use directional arrows and signs (toilets, dining room, lounge) to promote his independence and orientate him.

   ° Avoid contact with residents who 'wind' him up (e.g. Joe).

   ° When he 'follows' you this is a sign that he is anxious. On such occasions he seems to be missing his wife. Hence ask to see the picture of his wife he keeps in his pocket, and tell him when she is visiting next.

   ° Try to engage him in activities he enjoys, such as: walks, watching videos of rugby games, playing bowls, looking at pictures of dogs and birds.

   ° Enable him to use past coping strategies – let him go for a walk until he's calmed down.

   ° He loves ice cream. If you think he is becoming distressed in the afternoon, offer him one.

   ° Give him attention when he is in a good mood; he enjoys physical contact at these times.

2. What to do when Gordon is already aroused or angry.

- ° If Gordon says no – he means NO! Back off – don't crowd him – don't shout, either at him or call for assistance, unless you feel you are in danger. Adopt a calm, friendly approach. Validate his feelings and ask if you can help. If he says no, keep a watchful eye on him at a distance until he calms down.

3. Assisting with personal care

- ° Look for 'windows' of opportunity for personal hygiene activities. Gordon has times when he is more amenable, which often provide the best opportunities. For example, after: a walk; an ice cream; a can of lager, or when he has sought you out for attention.

- ° Bathing is usually a time when Gordon feels overwhelmed. From our discussion with staff, Joan (qualified nurse) and Brian (care worker) have the greatest success with this activity. Therefore they will advise on approaches/tactics and they put this in Gordon's care plan.

It is relevant to note that these interventions are active treatment strategies that needed to be developed and tweaked over time. They were used on a trial and error basis, and evolve as further feedback and insight was gained by the staff.

Outcome

The problematic behaviours were not eliminated completely, but by addressing the needs that were driving Gordon's behaviour, the episodes of aggression were significantly reduced. He remained in the home and was neither admitted to hospital, nor transferred. His diazepam was reduced from 25 mg daily to 5 mg daily. In relation to the NPI, the score improved from 14 to 6 by the end of treatment.

Case 2: John

Reason for referral

John, aged 71 years, was referred by a consultant psychiatrist because of inappropriate sexual behaviour. John had a ten-year history of Parkinson's disease and now had severe intellectual and physical impairments and poor verbal communication abilities. He spent most of his time in his bed and had developed pressure sores. At the time of referral he had an eight-week history of 'excessive' masturbating, which the staff at the nursing home were finding difficult. He frequently ejaculated onto himself, his bed, and sometimes in public places.

Assessment

As one might imagine, staff were upset by this behaviour, as illustrated by the following quotes:

'It's not nice for the staff.'

'Thirty years nursing and I have not come across anything like this.'

'Isn't there a tablet to stop it?'

'If he doesn't stop it, he'll need to leave.'

'Staff should not have to put up with this behaviour.'

John's placement was under threat because of his BC. There appeared to be a lack of understanding of John's illness and staff knew little of his life history.

This referral presented as a crisis and so in order to reduce the risk of him being moved quickly, a first step was to 'buy' more time with the staff. This was done by asking for a list of volunteer staff who would be willing to care for him over the initial weeks of the intervention – shift patterns needed to be changed accordingly. This organisational change provided us with time to implement our work, but it also identified staff who were more motivated than the others to engage with John. During any intervention such staff are important to find because they often hold different attitudes and are frequently interacting better with the resident; a lot of learning and transferring of skills can be achieved by working through such staff.

Charts were completed for the behaviour, but few patterns seemed to emerge. For example, he masturbated three to four times over the course of the day. It did not appear to be triggered by anything or anybody in particular. He performed the act on his own, in front of others, and on one occasion during a visit from his grandchildren. Interestingly, unlike many cases of sexual disihibition, he rarely masturbated or became aroused during intimate personal care activities. This was an important factor to recognise because it suggested that John was not hyper-aroused, a situation occasionally treated with an anti-androgen (i.e. a drug for reducing libido).

His wife informed us that the BC was completely out of character, and that he had always been a shy man, but someone who liked to talk through things at great length. She said that whenever he had a problem, he used to worry a lot and liked sharing his concerns with others. She also told us that he was a very physical person, someone who always held your hand and enjoyed a 'good' hug. He was also an extremely active man, who liked running, cycling and long walks.

From discussions with the psychiatrist and from clinical observations it became apparent that John had frontal lobe deficits. Unfortunately, his poor speech prevented any formal neuropsychological assessment of this. However, we used the frontal observation tool (FOT, James 2009) introduced in Chapter 2 (see Table 2.9) to get some clues about his abilities; his scores are presented in Table 7.1. The results on the FOT were suggestive of major frontal difficulties, but the fact that many of the queries could not be answered because of his physical problems (i.e. the NAs) gave us an idea about how isolated this man was feeling.

For a summary of his background and further details about the BC see Figure 7.2. It is relevant to remember, that John could not communicate well verbally, so the staff had to make a 'best guess' about what he may have been thinking and feeling based on discussions occurring in the ISS.

Intervention

The focus of the intervention was to increase understanding and change staff attitudes towards John.

Instructions recorded in the Care Plan:

1. Staff training.

   All staff to receive training in the following three areas: (i) sexuality issues in dementia – reflecting on companionship and sexuality; (ii) frontal lobe functioning and its effects on behaviour; (iii) advanced Parkinson's disease and how this can make people feel trapped inside their bodies and minds, particularly when someone's communication abilities are poor.

2. Practical solutions.

   It is unlikely that the behaviour is going to stop completely, so ways need to found to: (i) preserve John's dignity; (ii) make the clearing-up of the semen less unpleasant for the staff; (iii) provide opportunities for positive interactions with staff.

   i. Dignity – put a sheet over the cot sides to cover him and maintain his dignity when masturbating.
      John spends a lot of time in his bed wearing only a pyjama top and a continence pad. He often fiddles with the pad, which may be prompting his touching of his penis. When possible help him to wear loose fitting trousers, and encourage him to sit in his wheel-chair and get out of his room.

   ii. Cleaning up semen – encourage him to masturbate inside a pillow-case, which can be removed once he's ejaculated. Keep hand-wipes close to his bed, and encourage him to clean his hands regularly.

   iii. Positive interactions with staff – John likes physical contact and therefore give him a daily arm massage using aromatherapy oils – there is evidence that Melissa oil is helpful for people who are agitated.

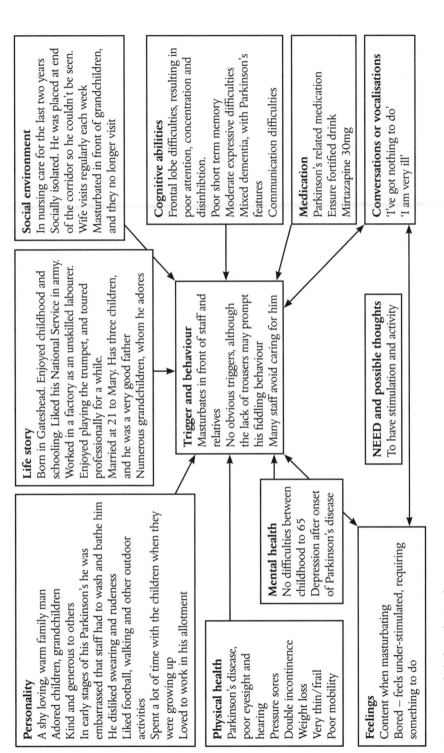

Social environment
In nursing care for the last two years
Socially isolated. He was placed at end
of the corridor so he couldn't be seen.
Wife visits regularly each week
Masturbated in front of grandchildren,
and they no longer visit

Cognitive abilities
Frontal lobe difficulties, resulting in
poor attention, concentration and
disinhibition.
Poor short term memory
Moderate expressive difficulties
Mixed dementia, with Parkinson's
features
Communication difficulties

Medication
Parkinson's related medication
Ensure fortified drink
Mirtazapine 30mg

Conversations or vocalisations
'I've got nothing to do'
'I am very ill'

Life story
Born in Gateshead. Enjoyed childhood and
schooling. Liked his National Service in army.
Worked in a factory as an unskilled labourer.
Enjoyed playing the trumpet, and toured
professionally for a while.
Married at 21 to Mary. Has three children,
and he was a very good father
Numerous grandchildren, whom he adores

Trigger and behaviour
Masturbates in front of staff and
relatives
No obvious triggers, although
the lack of trousers may prompt
his fiddling behaviour
Many staff avoid caring for him

NEED and possible thoughts
To have stimulation and activity

Personality
A shy loving, warm family man
Adored children, grandchildren
Kind and generous to others
In early stages of his Parkinson's he was
embarrassed that staff had to wash and bathe him
He disliked swearing and rudeness
Liked football, walking and other outdoor
activities
Spent a lot of time with the children when they
were growing up
Loved to work in his allotment

Physical health
Parkinson's disease,
poor eyesight and
hearing
Pressure sores
Double incontinence
Weight loss
Very thin/frail
Poor mobility

Mental health
No difficulties between
childhood to 65
Depression after onset
of Parkinson's disease

Feelings
Content when masturbating
Bored – feels under-stimulated, requiring
something to do

Figure 7.2 John's formulation sheet

Table 7.2 John's score on the FOT: an observation tool for assessing frontal functioning

Difficulties	Practical description of difficulty	John's score (1–5: not like him – to – totally like him)
Poor short-term/ working memory	Unable to correctly remember things done during the present day (e.g. breakfast, activities, etc.).	5
Recognition of objects, but unaware how to use them	Able to name an object, but unable to demonstrate its use (e.g. able to name a fork, but not aware how to use it)	NA – communication problems
Overly fixated on people or activities	Repeatedly paying attention, talking about or touching things (people, objects). Repetitive actions or activities.	4
Poor at making decisions	Unable to make choices, or decisions about what to do next (e.g. the person can't decide what he wants to wear or is unable to choose his food at meal times)	NA – ? not mobile
Poor planning	Unable to work out how to tackle a problem. For example, when a difficulty arises the client doesn't know where to begin, or can't grasp the nature of the problems (e.g. failing to move items off a table, before putting new ones on; doesn't recognise it would be helpful to write out a shopping list prior to going shopping)	4

Poor sequencing	Unable to carry out actions in a logical sequence (e.g. unable to dress themselves in a logical order, or when toileting tend to open bowels prior to removing underwear).	4
Concrete thinking	Unable to think in an abstract way. Conversations tend to be interpreted in an overly direct manner (If told *'it will all come out in the wash'*, he/she thinks this refers to washing clothes)	NA – unable to tell
Confabulation	Prone to giving stories and/or explanations in order to fill in gaps in his/her memory	NA
Lack of insight	Unaware of his current difficulties and limitations. Not being aware of the risks associated with these limitations (e.g. failing to appreciate he would not be able to live by himself at home)	3
Poor concentration	Unable to concentrate on anything for an extended period of time (e.g. watching TV, reading). Client's focus tends to move quickly on to something else	5
Distractibility	Easily distracted by things going on in the environment. When undertaking a task will lose interest in the task if interrupted by someone of something (e.g. a sound).	4
Perseveration	Repeating actions and statements over and over again	5
Unable to inhibit responses	Unable to control aggressive or sexual actions/statements that would be out of character from premorbid personality	5

Table 7.2 John's score on the FOT: an observation tool for assessing frontal functioning cont.

Difficulties	Practical description of difficulty	John's score (1–5: not like him – to – totally like him)
Saying things to hurt feelings	Making unkind comments about others which can serve to provoke or upset them.	NA
Impulsive actions and emotions	Suddenly doing something dangerous or risky – 'out of the blue'. Sudden outbursts of emotion	3
Emotionally flat	Emotionally unresponsive, even when being provoked	5 – bored
Euphoria	Overly enthusiastic, and/or inappropriately laughing out loud	1

3. Dealing with John's boredom.

John appears bored a lot of the time. Because of his behaviour, he is often left alone in his room. His boredom may be a key reason for his masturbating. It is important to help him get out of his room, and interact more with others. The staff have suggested the following activities.

   i. Encourage staff and family to take him outside of the home – some preparations will be required. For example, when dressing to go outside in his wheel-chair, ask him to wear tie-string trousers, making it more difficult for him to touch his penis. He could also be encouraged to wear mittens or gloves, which are also likely to discourage his 'fiddling'. Also, John is right handed and therefore someone taking him out could hold his right hand during the trip. John enjoys holding people's hand.

   ii. When washing him in the bath, ask him to hold items (soap, shampoo) so both hands are occupied.

Once staff were spending more time with him, rather than avoiding him, it became apparent that he did not masturbate when he was sitting up in his chair. One of the staff had the helpful idea of sitting him in his chair when his family visited. This plan was a great success, and his family began to visit on a regular basis again. The staff who had agreed to work with John during the first few weeks, also provided the rest of the staff with some good guidance. The most helpful observation was that John would stop masturbating when told to. However, he needed to be reminded every few minutes due to his memory problems, but he would comply if he was repeatedly prompted.

Outcome

Following the intervention, there was a moderate reduction in his behaviour. The main change occurred in staff's attitudes. As expressed in this quote, 'It is normal, we'll have to get on with it.' The practical solutions gave the staff a greater sense of control, and even those staff who were still upset by his behaviour no longer blamed him. John was no longer 'a dirty old man', but a man who was 'lonely and bored, with a habit he couldn't control'.

The scores on the NPI were 10 and 7 pre- and post respectively. Note the relatively small change on the behavioural scores, but the larger movement in terms of carer distress scores from 15 to 5.

Case 3: Isabel

Reason for referral

Isabel, aged 87, was referred from the elderly psychiatric ward where she had been admitted 5 months previously. She had been diagnosed with schizophrenia 12 years ago and had been admitted to hospital numerous times since then. She was currently experiencing auditory hallucinations with derogatory contents and was presenting with self-hitting behaviour. It was noted that Isabel's self-hitting behaviour increased when she was stressed.

Assessment

Isabel slapped her face continuously during the first assessment visit. She said that she was hearing the voices of relatives asking her for money. She would respond 'No' to the voices, and she said that this would lead them to take control of her hand. Staff felt that Isabel had a degree of control over her behaviour. They thought she was using the behaviour to try to get more time in her room. When she was not allowed access to her room, her slapping behaviour would increase.

One of the most helpful aspects of this case was the attendance of her estranged daughter, Joan, at the ISS. Joan provided a view of her mother as a very rigid person, who functioned by using strict routines. We were told that Isabel had one friend throughout her life; someone who was pretty similar to herself. Joan described her father as being very protective towards her mother, and it was he who provided the parental love. It seems that Isabel very rarely showed any emotions and was unable to empathise with either her or her brother. These details were put together with information from the staff, who on reflection, described Isabel as a frightened individual, someone who often looked scared of the other patients. During the ISS some of the staff began to see that she may be slapping her face as a sign of her distress. Based on this change in perspective, they saw her BC as being driven by a need to feel secure, to have time alone and to have some control over her life. This information, together with other details gained over the assessment period, are presented in Figure 7.3.

As one can see from the diagram in Figure 7.3, it was suggested that Isabel had autistic traits. To support this hypothesis, I asked Joan to complete the Relatives' Autism Quotient (rAQ, Baron-Cohen et al. 2001). This is a relatives' version of the Autism Quotient, which has been used in a previous study to identify Asperger's syndrome in older people (James et al. 2006c). Epidemiological figures concerning the frequency of this condition in the general population (1:1000) suggests that it is also a relatively common condition in older people; although it is grossly under-diagnosed. The results from the rAQ were consistent with someone with Asperger's syndrome.

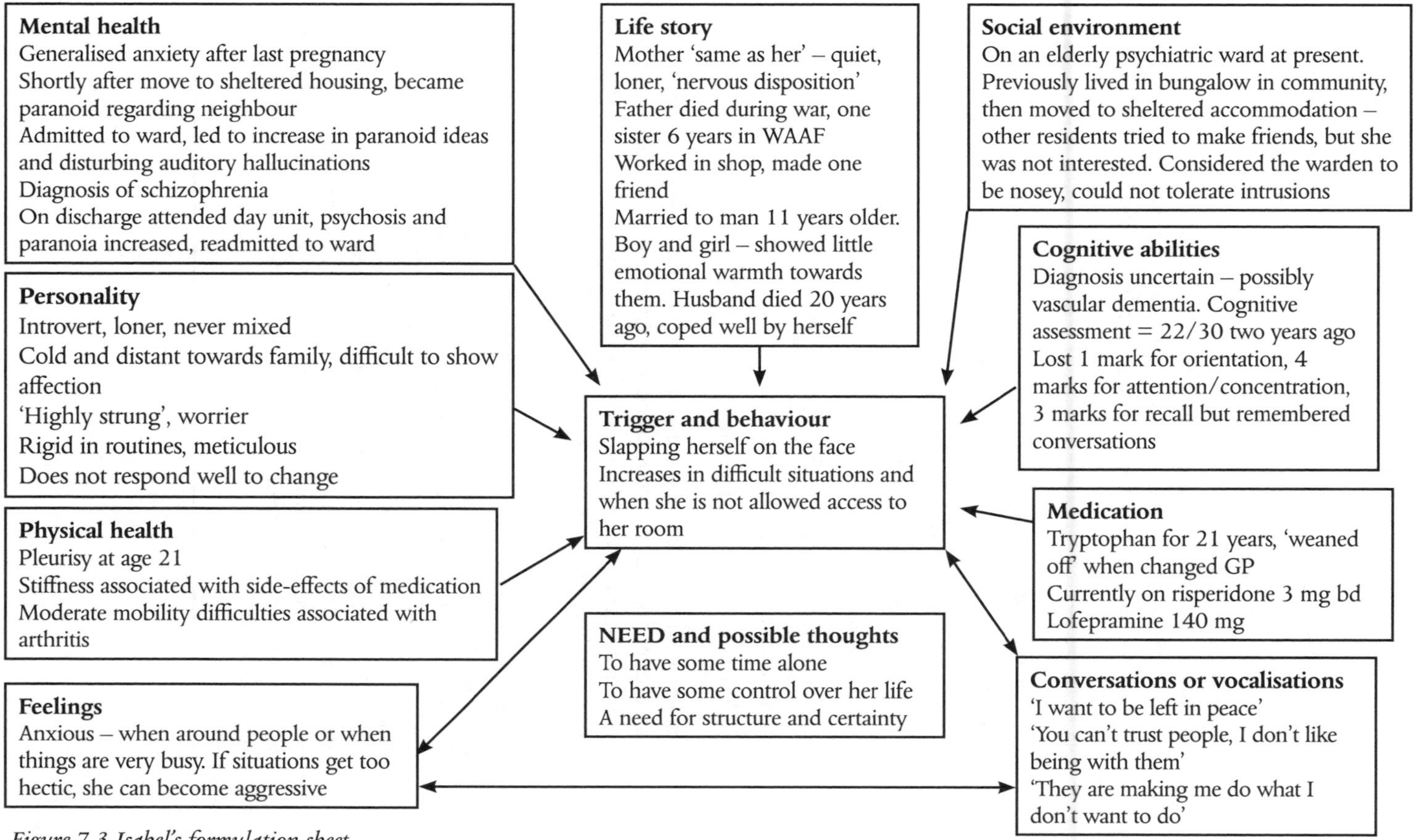

Mental health

Generalised anxiety after last pregnancy. Shortly after move to sheltered housing, became paranoid regarding neighbour. Admitted to ward, led to increase in paranoid ideas and disturbing auditory hallucinations. Diagnosis of schizophrenia. On discharge attended day unit, psychosis and paranoia increased, readmitted to ward

Personality

Introvert, loner, never mixed. Cold and distant towards family, difficult to show affection. 'Highly strung', worrier. Rigid in routines, meticulous. Does not respond well to change

Physical health

Pleurisy at age 21. Stiffness associated with side-effects of medication. Moderate mobility difficulties associated with arthritis

Feelings

Anxious – when around people or when things are very busy. If situations get too hectic, she can become aggressive

Life story

Mother 'same as her' – quiet, loner, 'nervous disposition'. Father died during war, one sister 6 years in WAAF. Worked in shop, made one friend. Married to man 11 years older. Boy and girl – showed little emotional warmth towards them. Husband died 20 years ago, coped well by herself

Trigger and behaviour

Slapping herself on the face. Increases in difficult situations and when she is not allowed access to her room

NEED and possible thoughts

To have some time alone. To have some control over her life. A need for structure and certainty

Social environment

On an elderly psychiatric ward at present. Previously lived in bungalow in community, then moved to sheltered accommodation – other residents tried to make friends, but she was not interested. Considered the warden to be nosey, could not tolerate intrusions

Cognitive abilities

Diagnosis uncertain – possibly vascular dementia. Cognitive assessment = 22/30 two years ago. Lost 1 mark for orientation, 4 marks for attention/concentration, 3 marks for recall but remembered conversations

Medication

Tryptophan for 21 years, 'weaned off' when changed GP. Currently on risperidone 3 mg bd. Lofepramine 140 mg

Conversations or vocalisations

'I want to be left in peace'. 'You can't trust people, I don't like being with them'. 'They are making me do what I don't want to do'

Figure 7.3 Isabel's formulation sheet

Intervention

Once it was clear that Isabel had Asperger's, it became evident that the intervention needed to be extremely structured, mimicking the rigidity and routines she had used throughout her life. This required negotiations with all the ward staff to permit Isabel to operate via different schedules to other patients; initially this approach met with much opposition.

The specific plan was to reduce Isabel's level of distress by meeting her need for routine and structure. This was done by negotiating times with the staff when she could be by herself in her room. An example of a timetable that was negotiated successfully is provided below.

Dining room Breakfast before 10.00 am and medication

Own room   10.15 am – 11.45 am

Dining room 11.45 am – 2.00 pm

Own room   2.00 pm – 5.00 pm

Dining room 5.00 pm – 6.00 pm

Own room   6.00 pm – 8.00 pm – come out ready for bed

Dining room 8.00 pm – 9.00 pm

Then own room until morning.

The key worker presented the information and the plan to the rest of the staff group. Some of the staff did not like the intervention, suggesting that we were rewarding 'bad' behaviour. It was only after providing a training session on 'autism' that the staff agreed to implement the plan consistently.

Outcome

The intervention improved the situation considerably, although the hitting did not stop completely. Further, over time Isabel seemed to feel she had more control over her life and would come out of her room to spend time with the other patients when she wanted to. After a further month she successfully moved into a residential facility, where she continues to live. As part of the discharge process from the ward, the plan devised in the hospital was discussed with the staff in the care home to ensure that the lessons learned in hospital were transferred. Her NPI scores improved from 22 to 10.

Case 4: Betsy
Reason for referral

Betsy, aged 85 years, was living with her husband in their own home. Stan, her husband, reported a number of problems, including her tendency to constantly follow him around. She had also recently hit a pregnant neighbour in the stomach, who was escorting her back to the house when Betsy became confused during a shopping trip. She appeared angry at times, clenching her fists and slapping Stan. Stan had responded to these difficulties by trying to keep his wife in the house, and taking over the running of the home.

Assessment

Betsy's BC was increasing and becoming more of a problem for Stan, who was struggling largely by himself. When charts were used to get a better understanding of his difficulties, it was evident that the situation was becoming critical. For example, Betsy had started to try to climb out of windows, and on one occasion had climbed on the ledge of a first floor window. Episodes of verbal aggression, slamming doors and refusing food and drink were recorded on the assessment charts.

Stan and his children were asked to arrange an ISS, and details were gathered about Betsy's background and her BC. Following the meeting, the family were provided with a summary of the information that had been discussed (see Figure 7.4).

Intervention

Discussion took place with staff about the nature of Betsy's cognitive difficulties. She had expressive dysphasia, so was struggling to communicate verbally, but her receptive dysphasia was only mild, so she was aware of what was being said to her. We used information about the cognitive triads to explain some of the difficult dynamics, and to help the children empathise better with their parents' situation (see Figure 7.5). At the end of the ISS, the family agreed on the following guidance for helping Betsy. The instructions recorded in the family plan were:

- Support Stan, as he is struggling to cope. He needs help from the family and additional support from social services.

- Watch out for and avoid triggers. Betsy does not like to hear raised voices and will become distressed if shouted at.

- Watch out for signs that she is going to become anxious. Typically the signs are when her speech becomes clearer, or she starts patting herself, or when she starts banging the windows.

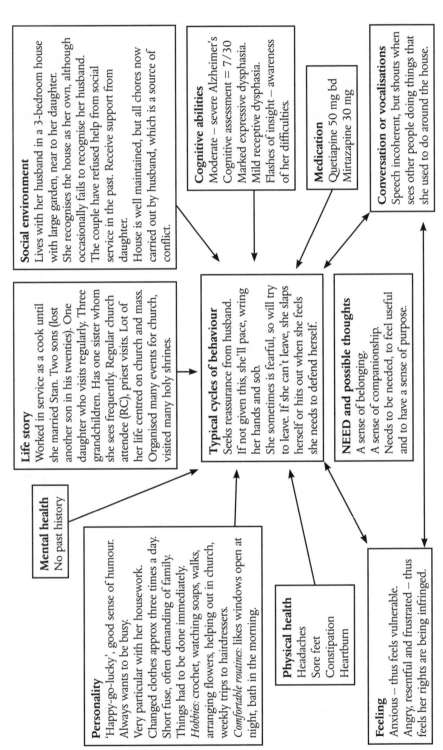

Social environment
Lives with her husband in a 3-bedroom house with large garden, near to her daughter.
She recognises the house as her own, although occasionally fails to recognise her husband.
The couple have refused help from social service in the past. Receive support from daughter.
House is well maintained, but all chores now carried out by husband, which is a source of conflict.

Cognitive abilities
Moderate – severe Alzheimer's
Cognitive assessment = 7/30
Marked expressive dysphasia.
Mild receptive dysphasia.
Flashes of insight – awareness of her difficulties.

Medication
Quetiapine 50 mg bd
Mirtazapine 30 mg

Conversation or vocalisations
Speech incoherent, but shouts when sees other people doing things that she used to do around the house.

Life story
Worked in service as a cook until she married Stan. Two sons (lost another son in his twenties). One daughter who visits regularly. Three grandchildren. Has one sister whom she sees frequently. Regular church attendee (RC), priest visits. Lot of her life centred on church and mass. Organised many events for church, visited many holy shrines.

Mental health
No past history

Typical cycles of behaviour
Seeks reassurance from husband.
If not given this, she'll pace, wring her hands and sob.
She sometimes is fearful, so will try to leave. If she can't leave, she slaps herself or hits out when she feels she needs to defend herself.

NEED and possible thoughts
A sense of belonging.
A sense of companionship.
Needs to be needed, to feel useful and to have a sense of purpose.

Personality
'Happy-go-lucky', good sense of humour.
Always wants to be busy.
Very particular with her housework.
Changed clothes approx three times a day.
Short fuse, often demanding of family.
Things had to be done immediately.
Hobbies: crochet, watching soaps, walks, arranging flowers, helping out in church, weekly trips to hairdressers.
Comfortable routine: likes windows open at night, bath in the morning.

Physical health
Headaches
Sore feet
Constipation
Heartburn

Feeling
Anxious – thus feels vulnerable.
Angry, resentful and frustrated – thus feels her rights are being infringed.

Figure 7.4 Betsy's formulation sheet

- Fix child-locks to the window frames.

- Maintain a calm approach to supporting Betsy, make good use of non-verbal language (e.g. smile, approach her slowly and be patient).

- Use distraction techniques if she is becoming anxious. For example, invite her to sit in her favourite chair and play her music tapes (hymns or Daniel O'Donnell). Encourage her to watch videos of church service, 'You've been Framed' or favourite soaps. Sit with her and read the Bible to her. Go out with her.

- Attempt to give her a sense of belonging. Thus rather than doing things for her, let her do things for herself. She is bound to make mistakes, but encourage her to be active and praise her for this. For example, encourage her to help out around the home (e.g. dusting, baking, washing and drying dishes, supervised cooking).

- Betsy loves cuddles; remember to be tactile and make use of this important sense that she retains. Let her see you understand that she's struggling, but you still love her.

Outcome

Betsy's behaviour became much more settled and her psychotropic medication was reduced significantly. Her family were able to predict when Betsy was becoming agitated and used the distraction techniques more successfully. Intervening at this earlier stage usually prevented Betsy's anxiety from increasing. Her scores on the NPI improved markedly from 28 to 5, and the caregiver distress score changed from 12 to 3.

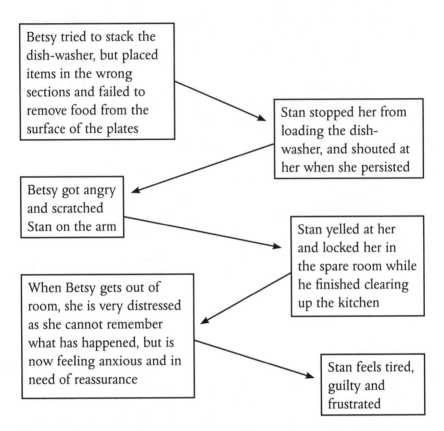

Figure 7.5 Typical example of a negative sequence occurring prior to the intervention

INTERVENTIONS USED BY THE NCBT

The case examples described above illustrate that the interventions are formulation-led and are individually tailored around the needs of the people with dementia. In 2009, Mackin undertook an audit of the interventions carried out by members of the NCBT. A table summarising her findings is presented in Table 7.3. She used Cohen-Mansfield's categorisation system (see Chapter 1) to distinguish between the various BC treated by the team; Table 7.3 presents the findings for the verbal agitation category of BC only (shouting, screaming, etc.).

Table 7.3 Summary of NCBT Interventions (Makin 2009)

Instrumental goal	Intervention theme
Stimulation	Improve communication Provide personalised activity Change in physical interpersonal interactions with client One-to-one time Provide explanation of action Ensure client is awake and alert prior to commencing interventions Gain permission to carry out action or enter personal space Therapeutic lie Orientation to people and environment Inform about repercussions of actions Distraction Arrange trip away from the home or ward
Comfort	Give client own space Simulation presence
Practical assistance	Minimise background noise Leave the area and return after a short period Provide medication (pain or anti-depressant) Client moved from distressing environment Provide drinks or food client likes Schedule regular toilet breaks
Status	Involve in work on the ward or at the home
Behavioural confirmation	Consistent approach from carers Promote independence Offer client choice (e.g. clothing or activity) Offer praise for action or attire Offer reassurance Reward positive behaviour verbally or with 'treats' Decrease number of choices – simplifying
Affection	Empathise with person's difficulties Use of physical affection (hold hand, hug) Doll therapy Personal video (family, pet, friend)

The table does not describe individual interventions, but summarises the data into themes. While this makes the data more manageable, some of the rich descriptiveness is clearly lost. Nevertheless, the reader can see that the strategies are a mix of person-focused and carer-centred interventions. Further, they are all 'needs-led', with the goals aimed at meeting basic human requirements for appropriate environments, companionship, acknowledgement, comfort and stimulation (Maslow 1943). The other key thing to note is that the interventions are relatively basic. They are chiefly concerned with improving communication and interpersonal skills, rather than with the initiation of complex psychological therapies. This is because of two main features; first, the approaches are often derived by the carers during the information sharing session. Second, many of the strategies employed are refined versions of partially successful strategies used by the carers previously. However, owing to the NCBT's clinical input, these very practical strategies can now be employed in tighter, better defined ways, with a high degree of consensus and consistency.

CONCLUSION

This chapter has examined case material from the work of the NCBT across various settings: care homes, hospitals and in people's own homes. Clearly, there are slight adaptations to the method of working within each place; although broadly speaking the basic processes remain the same. For example, in each case the BC is treated as a sign or symptom of some underlying issue, and the job of the therapist is to recruit the carers into a 'forensic' team capable of uncovering the causal factors. This forensic approach to BC is not unique to the NCBT, and examples of similar methodologies can be found elsewhere (Cohen-Mansfield *et al.* 2007; Bird *et al.* 2009). In relation to the interventions, it is evident that they are linked to the formulations and that they are devised with the assistance of the carers. As outlined in the previous chapter, it is essential that the carers have ownership of the strategies used. Further, as partners in this process, the carers are able to tweak the interventions as they see fit because they are clear about the rationales underpinning them.

Chapter 8

Service Development and Provision

INTRODUCTION

Major concerns about financial costs, services not being fit for purpose, over-use of medication, and so on, have resulted in calls for the development of new models of health and social care for people with challenging behaviours. The private sector must be included in such frameworks because the care homes look after 33 per cent of those diagnosed with dementia and such residents often have the most complex needs ('Remember, I'm still me; CC/MWC 2009). This chapter examines recent recommendations made by Banerjee (2009) about reforming services for the treatment of BC. The second part of the chapter provides details of the aims and structure of the Newcastle Challenging Behaviour Team (NCBT), which was established in 1999. By providing service related details of the team, other clinicians wishing to develop such services may learn from our experiences, both the successes and mistakes. The final section examines research studies undertaken by NCBT members. Their involvement in such work has helped to sustain their enthusiasm and motivation in an area often associated with staff burn-out.

By the end of this chapter the reader will be aware of the following:

- Banerjee (2009) has provided a number of useful recommendations relating to service development.

- Relatively small case-loads and regular supervision are essential features of the practice of a BC clinician.

- Working into different settings (care homes, wards, etc.) requires adjustments to how the clinical work is delivered.

- BC work is stressful and thus it is helpful for therapists working in the area to be engaged in other forms of service related activities (teaching, research, dissemination, etc.). Such work has additional benefits for the service and also for carers and families.

- Service related research is an important feature of a clinical team. It improves practical knowledge-bases, facilitates reflection and sustains morale.

SERVICE REFORM

Banerjee (2009) has set out a programme aimed at reducing the existing use of anti-psychotic medication for people with dementia by 66 per cent over a period of 36 months. In order to achieve this he made 11 recommendations, which dove-tail well with the objectives of the English and Scottish Dementia Strategies (2009, 2010). Most of Banerjee's recommendations are pertinent to this text, but the following three suggestions are the most relevant.

1. The commissioning of specialist services to work in care homes (Recommendation 8).

2. Improving carers' knowledge of non-pharmacological strategies (Recommendation 7).

3. The need for research on treatments for BC, particularly non-pharmacological strategies (Recommendation 5).

Each of these recommendations is outlined below in more detail.

Recommendation 8

Each primary care trust should commission from local specialist older people's mental health services an in-reach service that supports primary care in its work in care homes. This extension of service needs the capacity to work routinely in all care homes where there may be people with dementia. They may be aided by regular pharmacist input into homes. This is a core recommendation of this report and it requires new capacity to be commissioned by primary care trusts in order that the other recommendations can be met.

In this recommendation, he discusses the multi-disciplinary nature of such an in-reach service, and the need for it to be able to respond quickly in order to support care staff struggling with difficult behaviours. Banerjee thinks that it is essential to have good links with the local GPs, working with them in a coordinated manner. In his discussion of a service model, he suggests having specialist clinicians distributed within existing community mental health teams (CMHTs); this is in preference to having stand-alone specialist teams. In Australia, Brodaty *et al.* (2003) proposed introducing a triangular model for the organisation and services for BC. It is a seven tiered pyramid with the higher levels denoting lower prevalence but greater severity of behaviour. They suggest that people can move and down the tiers (e.g. aggression occurring due to an infection, may reduce as the infection is treated), and the service provision will track the changes. This model has been influential in developing service policy.

Recommendation 7

There is a need to develop a curriculum for the development of appropriate skills for care home staff in the non-pharmacological treatment of behavioural disorder in dementia, including the deployment of specific therapies with positive impact. Senior staff in care homes should have these skills and the ability to transfer them to other staff members in care homes. A national vocational qualification in dementia care should be developed for those working with people with dementia.

It was noted that care homes are now managing many more complex residents compared to 30 years ago; with higher concentrations of people with multiple physical and cognitive needs. Banerjee, supporting the findings of the All-Party Parliamentary Report on Dementia (2008), highlights that there are currently major deficiencies in the knowledge, attitude and skills amongst carers. As a result he suggests that the Department of Health work with training organisations to develop National Vocational Qualifications in Dementia Care for those working in care settings. It is worth noting that he also calls for improvements in the skill bases of GPs, psychiatrists and other professionals (Schols *et al.* 2004). Under Recommendation 7, Banerjee outlines some of the potential non-pharmacological strategies that staff should be trained in on their various courses. Unfortunately, this section is short on detail, and remains an area requiring more attention if non-pharmacological approaches are to be presented as realistic alternatives to medication.

Recommendation 5

There is a need for further research to be completed, including work assessing the clinical and cost effectiveness of non-pharmacological methods of treating behavioural problems in dementia and of other pharmacological approaches as an alternative to anti-psychotic medication. The National Institute for Health Research and the Medical Research Council should work to develop programmes of work in this area.

There are gaps in the evidence-base for all the proposed treatments, but this is a particular concern for non-pharmacological strategies if they are to be used as the first-line alternative to psychotropics. There is clearly a case for large randomised controlled trials in this area, but there is also the need for process-research that describes in detail how to implement some of the psychological methodologies put forward in the existing national guidelines (e.g. NICE guidelines for dementia).

Recent years have seen the development of a number of well-funded large scale programmes. Examples include; Challenge-Demcare (Moniz-Cook *et al.* 2008c) and WHELD (Ballard *et al.* Alzheimer's Society 2010). The former is an interactive web-based system that guides clinicians and carers to develop care plans. The features of the program provide education and training in the assessment and tailoring of person-centred interventions. The treatment approach itself is firmly grounded in functional analysis (FA), with all aspects of the program linked overtly to FA (assessment, conceptualisation, treatment). WHELD seeks to develop an evidence-based treatment guide based on a component analysis of previous interventions that have been shown to work. The first stage of this five year study has been to undertake an extensive literature review of qualitative and quantitative studies conducted in the area. Important innovative work is also being undertaken by Brooker and colleagues in a programme called PEARL, which utilises a development of Dementia Care Mapping called VIPS (Brooker, 2007).

The following section presents an example of an established BC service that fulfils many of the recommendations outlined in Banerjee's report, although it is a stand-alone service rather than being embedded within a larger mental health team.

DESCRIPTION OF THE DEVELOPMENT AND WORK OF THE NEWCASTLE CHALLENGING BEHAVIOUR TEAM (NCBT)

Before providing details of the NCBT, it is worth highlighting that there are a number of well-established teams across the UK, undertaking similar work to Newcastle's. Four of the most notable are the Northern Irish (Homefirst), Sutton, Doncaster and Gloucester liaison teams. The NCBT is one of three similar teams in the North East of England. It was the first community BC team in the region, established in 2000. The other teams are part of the same NHS Trust but operate differently owing to geography and staff composition. For example, the Northumberland County BC team covers a very large rural area and by necessity works very closely with the community mental health teams in the localities. The South of Tyne BC team, unlike the other services, does not have any clinical psychology input and is composed of nurses and occupational therapists. All three services are specialist stand-alone teams and use the same basic biopsychosocial methodology outlined in Chapter 6.

Details of the populations covered by the three BC teams are provided in Table 8.1.

Table 8.1 Demographics for areas in North East England that have BC teams

Area (2007 – NTW* NHS Trust figures)	Population of 65+	Percentage of over 65s, aged 85+	Cases of dementia
England	8168.8K	13.3	595,000
Newcastle	41K	13.4	3050
Northumberland	58.5K	12.1	4080
Sunderland and South Tyneside	72.9K	21.9	4960

* Northumberland Tyne and Wear NHS Foundation Trust.

Currently the NCBT is made-up of two senior nurses and four mid-grade nurses. It is managed by a consultant clinical psychologist and receives sessional input from a consultant psychiatrist. Over the last decade, 1400+ people have received interventions using this approach; currently the NCBT sees approximately 200 community clients per year, and works onto a 20-bedded dementia inpatient unit.

The original reason for establishing the Newcastle team was because of a gap in the existing clinical services in the locality for people living in care. This meant that some of the most complex people in our communities were not receiving adequate psychological care. Traditionally, the private sector care homes had proven difficult places to work into, because they had not previously received sustained attention from health service psychotherapists. Thus they were rather wary of input when it was offered. They tended to prefer medication over therapy, owing to the clinical commitments the latter entailed. Due to the poor reception received, previously NHS therapists had been reluctant to engage with these settings (James, Powell and Kendell 2003b). In order to break this negative cycle, the NCBT was established, with the following aims:

- to treat BC in a competent and carer-centred, person-focused manner
- to provide a biopsychosocial model of care in which pharmacological and non-pharmacological interventions were given as part of a rational treatment plan
- to treat BC in the setting in which they are exhibited because the settings are often linked to the behaviours
- to work collaboratively with care facilities to improve the well-being of people in care
- to prevent unnecessary admissions to hospital
- to facilitate effective discharges from hospital to appropriate care settings
- to facilitate transfers of patients to appropriate care settings (from hospital to care facilities and between care facilities)
- to develop links with statutory and regulatory organizations (e.g. Care Quality Commission).

Working into care homes can be extremely stressful work, especially when the therapist is trying to avoid the unnecessary use of medication in favour of non-pharmacological approaches. Thus clinician burn-out is a constant risk. To prevent this happening, each NCBT member's case load is small (n = 10–12). The staff are also provided with frequent supervision (minimum of 1 hour per week), and they operate within a separate specialist team from a single centre. The latter allows for support and permits informal supervision as and when required. While the clinical work is the core task of the team, the therapists partake in non-clinical activities. The extra activities are outlined in Figure 8.1 and involve teaching, consultancy and research.

While the teaching is seen as an essential element of the clinical work of the team (i.e. teaching care staff), the requirement to constantly update presentations ensures that the team members keep themselves up-to-date with new developments in the area. Research is also viewed as an important feature of the NCBT. However, it has been agreed with management that all projects need to address clinical issues relating directly to service delivery. Examples of some of the resulting projects are outlined in the next section.

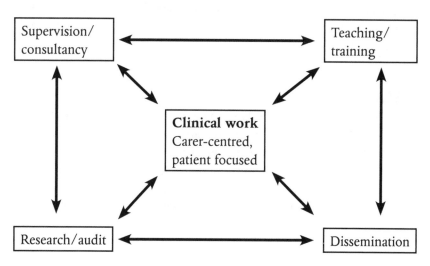

Figure 8.1 NCBT activity grid (Mackenzie 2008)

In recent years, and in keeping with the recommendations made within the National Dementia Strategies, the NCBT has started to work more consistently into the local dementia inpatient unit. The basic clinical model used in this setting is similar to that used in the community (i.e. helping staff to disengage emotionally and obtain more factual information about the person with dementia and the BC), but the methodology has changed to meet the needs of the setting (see Dexter-Smith 2010). It is worth noting that earlier attempts to operate on the inpatient unit had met with difficulties because ward staff appeared to find it difficult to fit the formulation process into existing formats used by the wards. Another major problem had been the variations in practice of the different consultant psychiatrists working onto the ward. Latterly, such difficulties have been tackled by a reconfiguration of the service. In the new service there is only one consultant psychiatrist for the ward and he holds regular daily meetings attended routinely by a member of the NCBT.

As noted earlier in Chapter 7, empirical evaluation of the work of the NCBT has demonstrated its efficacy (Wood-Mitchell *et al.* 2007b, and see Chapter 6). It is suggested that the reasons for its success are to do with its values and desire to empower all people involved in dealing with the 'problematic' behaviours (i.e. the resident, staff, family, care home manager). This systemic stance helps to ensure that the formulation-led care plans are initiated and adhered to appropriately.

The next section illustrates some of the research and audits undertaken by members of the team. As Banerjee points out in his report, research is crucial for the development of the field.

RESEARCH

Each member of the NCBT is encouraged to conduct research as per Figure 8.1. It is expected that this research will form the basis of either a publication or a conference presentation. The nurses are supported in their endeavours by me and colleagues at Newcastle and Teesside Universities. In this section, a few of the interesting projects and research programmes are presented. Many of the other studies have been referred to in earlier sections of this book.

Toilet study

Stokes (2001) describes the difficulties many people with dementia have with using cold, smelly inhospitable toilets in care settings. He believes that because the toilet rooms/cubicles are rather unsavoury places, people are reluctant to use them and this may eventually lead to them becoming incontinent.

In order to highlight this issue, and get staff to reflect on what they themselves would need and expect before using a public toilet, we conducted a survey on toileting habits (Mackenzie 2004; James *et al.* 2007). In this survey staff were asked to state the various idiosyncratic habits they routinely employ when using a public WC. They chose from a checklist and were invited to provide details of their own habits. Some key findings are outlined in Table 8.2.

This study was really a vehicle for getting care staff to reflect on the difficulties that people with dementia have in using the toilets in care facilities. Indeed by getting carers to empathise with the residents and clients, it was thought that the staff would be armed with the knowledge and motivation to change their toileting practices and improve the 'user-friendliness' of the cubicles in terms of cleanliness, smells, and ergonomics. In addition, it was hoped that the research would increase staff's awareness of the important roles that privacy, dignity and autonomy play in maintaining people's comfort about using toilets. Finally, it was hoped that those participating in the study would be prompted to move from a 'task-focused' perspective, to one in which they saw toileting as a opportunity to demonstrate good care and respect. The next phase of this study will look at the impact of the staff's 'new-awareness' on their actual practices.

Doll therapy

Dolls have been used widely as a preventative therapy to promote feelings of well-being with people with dementia who are agitated or distressed, have communication difficulties, or are withdrawn (Godfrey 1994; Ehrenfeld 2003; Mayers 2003). Several anecdotal reports and case studies have found various types of 'life-like' baby dolls (e.g. raggy dolls, empathy dolls, 'Emily' dolls) to be effective for reducing agitation, aggression and wandering (e.g. Moore 2001; Gibson 2005).

In Newcastle, the NCBT have introduced dolls into a number of care settings and have conducted several studies investigating the impact of dolls on the residents who choose to use them. We have also produced guidelines for the use of dolls based on clinical observations (Mackenzie, Wood-Mitchell and James 2007). In the Mackenzie *et al.* study (2006), we found that 69 per cent of care staff reported improvement in residents' well-being. Specifically, they noted improvements in resident interaction with staff; interaction with other residents; level of activity; happiness/ contentment; amenability to care interventions and agitation. However,

Table 8.2 Summary of responses to the question 'Do you engage in any of the following activities when using a toilet which is not in your home?'

Activity	Always	Sometimes	Very occasionally	Never
Do you squat to avoid making contact with the toilet seat?	32.6%	38.0%	13.0%	16.3%
Would you place toilet paper on the seat if you have to sit on it?	38.0%	22.8%	12.0%	27.2%
Would you wipe round the toilet seat prior to using it?	46.2%	37.4%	8.8%	7.7%
Would you avoid touching the flush handle by using paper or another part of your anatomy?	25.3%	30.8%	17.6%	26.4%
When washing you hands, do you avoid touching the taps by using your wrists to turn taps on and off?	16.5%	27.5%	17.6%	38.5%
On leaving the toilet do you avoid touching the door handle?	20.9%	26.4%	15.4%	37.4%

the individual profiles varied greatly and the care staff reported some problems using the dolls (e.g. disputes over ownership, dolls being mislaid). Another of our studies (James, Mackenzie and Mukaetova-Ladinska 2006a) examined the use of dolls over a 12-week period and found that the majority of residents who chose to use a doll obtained some benefits on levels of activity, interaction with staff and other residents, happiness and agitation. Additionally, in the Ellingford *et al.* (2007) study we found that those people who chose to use a doll showed an increase in positive behaviour and a decrease in negative behaviour and incidents of aggression three months after the introduction of dolls.

The qualitative study by Fraser (Fraser and James 2008) suggested that the dolls met a range of basic 'needs' of those choosing to use them. These needs included attachment, comfort, activity, inclusion, communication/interaction, identity, memory and fantasy. It is, thus, hypothesised that the doll may offer an opportunity to deal with ongoing inner psychological distress in a more adaptive way. The latest study in this research programme is investigating the views of people with dementia in settings where dolls are regularly used. This work includes the opinions of doll users (Alander 2010).

From this entire body of work it appears that a doll can play a number of roles for the person with dementia. However, it is paramount that the doll use is guided by the person (Mackenzie, Wood-Mitchell and James 2007).

Use of lies in the care of people with dementia

Lying and deception are generally viewed as morally wrong (Vrij 2000), and can jeopardise the trust in relationships (DePaulo, Kashy *et al.* 1996). However, lies and deception play an important and complicated role in daily interactions. Lies can be told in the interests of others, preventing awkwardness and unnecessary rudeness. Vrij (2000) differentiated between: 'subtle lying' and 'exaggerations' and 'outright lying' (whereby the information communicated is contradictory or completely different to the truth). These categories are similar to those described in the dementia care literature. Blum (1994) found that family members of people with dementia considered 'outright lies' to be distinct from other forms of deception ('going along', 'little white lies', 'not telling', and 'tricks'). Indeed, Cunningham (2005) found that professional carers used euphemistic expressions (e.g. 'little white lies' and 'bending the truth') to reduce the inner conflicts associated with lying.

In Newcastle, we began to examine the use of lying by carers in 2002, and have since conducted a number of studies on the topic (James *et al.* 2003d, 2006d; Wood-Mitchell *et al.* 2007a; Elvish *et al.* 2010). Some of the key findings are outlined below.

- In a survey of 112 professional carers and therapists, 98 per cent of people admitted to telling lies to people with dementia.

- 93 per cent of participants thought lying could be beneficial.

- 88 per cent of participants acknowledged lies could be problematic.

- 85 per cent of participants wanted guidelines on the use of lies in dementia care.

- A number of studies have endorsed the view that lies should only be told in people with dementia's best interests.

- People with dementia acknowledge the potential benefits and problems of lying.

- People consider this is an important issue for debate because, whatever one thinks about the topic, lying is endemic in our care services.

The most recent study on this topic examined the views of people with dementia (Waterworth *et al.* in press). From this project it was recommended that carers should adopt a 'cautious' approach when utilising lies and deception. Most participants considered it to be more acceptable to use lying during the later stages of their dementia, because the benefits (a reduction of truth-related distress) were considered to outweigh the detractions (e.g. negative impact on personhood and self-esteem). However, several participants considered lying to be unacceptable under any circumstances.

In response to carers' requests for guidelines we have produced a 12-item guide (James *et al.* 2006d). One of the most controversial items is a suggestion that staff should be trained in the use of lies (e.g. choosing an appropriate lie, or how to document a lie, etc.). It is important to say that within this body of work we have never said that we endorse lying; however, we feel it is unethical to ignore this issue. It is apparent that staff and families view lying as part of their armoury of communication strategies, and they are often proud of the effectiveness of their lies in reducing distress in the person with dementia.

Other studies

In the recent past we have conducted many studies, tending to choose themes relating to practical issues – particularly to problems we have encountered while attempting to deliver care. A typical example of this is Smith's survey on the 'poor communication skills of carers whose first language is not English' (Smith *et al.* 2008). Another controversial topic concerns our investigation of sexuality issues relating to people with dementia and their carers. Currently our largest research programme involves asking carers' about their perceptions of the use of medication in BC.

In the last ten years the NCBT have published over 30 articles, writing in both peer-reviewed (60%) and non-reviewed journals. As one can see from the examples, the research is practical, relating directly to clinical issues encountered when working with people with dementia and their carers. We have forged good links with the local universities and work symbiotically with graduates requiring research projects as part of their courses. This relationship means that we can conduct studies without funding, and get help from the university staff with the issues involved in obtaining ethical approval. As a clinical team, we think it is vital that we undertake such practical research, and although the studies are often of a modest scale, the findings always relate directly to 'hands-on' clinical work.

CONCLUSION

This new century has seen the launch of important documents that will shape services that we are all likely to encounter as we move towards our own retirements, and beyond. While this is an incentive to improve care, we should also be motivated by the fact that older people, and particularly those with dementia, have received comparatively little strategically-guided attention in the past. The various UK National Dementia Strategies promise much, but it is going to be interesting to see what they actually deliver in the long term. Thus it is important that we attend to the on-going audits regarding the implementation of their proposals.

In relation to my own work, I think it is important to continue to develop models of care that are informed by theory and supported by audit and research. In this chapter, and within this book, I have presented the work of a team that is grounded in the 'scientist–practitioner' tradition, and that has evolved to meet the ever changing requirements of the NHS and private sector.

References

Alander, H. (2010) *Older Adults' Views and Experiences of Doll Therapy in Everyday Dementia Care.* Teesside University, Middlesbrough. DClinPsych Thesis.

Alexopoulos, G.S., Abrams, R.C., Young, R.C. and Shamoian, C.A. (1988) 'Cornell scale for depression in dementia'. *Biological Psychiatry 23*, 271–284.

Algase, D.L., *et al.* (1996) 'Need-driven dementia compromised behaviour: an alternative view of disruptive behavior'. *American Journal of Alzheimer's Disease and Other Dementias 11*, 10–19.

Alessi, C.A., Yoon, E.J., Schnelle, J.F., Al-Samarrai, N.R. and Cruise, P.A. (1999) 'A randomized trial of a combined physical activity and environmental intervention in nursing home residents: do sleep and agitation improve?' *Journal of the American Geriatric Society 47*, 7, 784–791.

Allen-Burge, R., Stevens, A. and Burgio, I. (1999) 'Effective behavioural interventions for decreasing dementia related challenging-behaviour in nursing homes'. *International Journal of Geriatric Psychiatry 14*, 213–232.

All-Party Parliamentary Group on Dementia (2008) 'Always a last resort: Inquiry into the prescription of antipsychotic drugs to people with dementia living in care homes'. April. www. Alzheimers.org.uk (accessed 15/06/2008).

Alzheimer's society (2010) Research e-journal issue 11: scientific version. Availaible at www. alzheimers.org.uk.

Ashida, S. (2002) 'The effect of reminiscence music therapy sessions on changes in depressive symptoms in elderly persons with dementia'. *Journal of Music Therapy 37*, 170–182.

Audit Commission (2002) *Forget me not.* www.audit-commission.gov.uk

Baker, R., Bell, S., Baker, E., *et al.* (2001) 'A randomised controlled trials of the effects of multi-sensory simulation for people with dementia'. *British Journal of Clinical Psychology 40*, 81–96.

Ballard, C., O'Brien, J., James, I., Swann, A. (2001) *Managing Behavioural and Psychological Symptoms in People with Dementia.* Oxford: Oxford University Press.

Ballard, C. Gauthier, S. Cummings, L., *et al.* (2009) 'Management of agitation and aggression associated with Alzheimer's disease'. *Nature Review (Neurology) 5*, 5, 245–255.

Ballard, C.G., O'Brien, J.T., Reichelt, K. and Perry, E.K. (2002) 'Aromatherapy as a safe and effective treatment for the management of agitation in severe dementia: The results of a double-blind, placebo-controlled trial with Melissa'. *Journal of Clinical Psychiatry 63*, 7, 553–558.

Banerjee, S. (2009) *The Use of Antipsychotic Medication for People with Dementia: Time for Action.* London: DoH.

Baron-Cohen, S. Wheelwright, S. and Skinner, R.I. (2001) 'The autism-spectrum quotient'. *Journal of Autism and Developmental Disorders 31*, 5–12.

Barber, N. (2009) 'Medication errors in care homes'. PSRP Briefing Paper, PSO25. University of Birmingham.

Beck, A.T. (1976) *Cognitive Therapy and the Emotional Disorders.* New York: International University Press.

Bird, M., Llwellyn-Jones, R.H., Korten, A. and Smithers, H. (2007) 'A controlled trial of a predominantly psychosocial approach to BPSD: Treating causality'. *International Psychogeriatrics 19*, 5, 874–891.

Bird, M., Llwellyn-Jones, R.H. and Korten, A. (2009) 'An evaluation of the effectiveness of a case-specific approach to challenging behaviour associate with dementia'. *Aging and Mental Health 13*, 1, 73–83.

Bishara, D., Taylor, D., Howard, R. and Abdel-Tawab, R. *et al.* (2009) 'Expert opinion on the management of BPSD and investigation into prescribing practices in the UK'. *International Journal of Geriatric Psychiatry 24*, 9, 944–954.

Blum, N.S. (1994) 'Deceptive practices in managing a family member with Alzheimer's disease'. *Symbolic Interaction 17*, 1, 21–36.

Blunden, R. and Allen, D. (1987) *Facing the Challenge: An Ordinary Life for People with Learning Difficulties and Challenging Behaviour.* London: King's Fund.

Bohlmeijer, E., Smit, F. and Cuipers, P. (2003) 'Effects of reminiscence and life review on late-life depression: a metal-analysis'. *International Journal of Geriatric Psychiatry 18*, 1088–1094.

Brodaty, H., Green, A. and Koschera, A. (2003) 'Meta-analysis of psychosocial interventions for caregivers of people with dementia'. *Journal of American Geriatric Society 51*, 657–664.

Brooker, D. (2006) 'Dementia care mapping: a review of the research literature'. *The Gerontologist 45*, 1, 11–18.

Brooker, D. (2007) *Person-Centred Dementia Care: Making Services Better.* London: Jessica Kingsley.

Burns, A. (2010). 'Editorial. Special issue: the challenges of dementia an international perspective'. *International Journal of Geriatric Psychiatry 25*, 9, 875.

Burns, A., Lawlor, B. and Craig, S. (1999) *Assessment Scales in Old Age Psychiatry.* London: Martin Dunitz.

Care Commission and Mental Welfare Commission (CC/MWC) (2009) *Remember, I'm Still Me: Care Commission and Mental Welfare Commission Joint Report on the Quality of Care of People with Dementia Living in Care Homes in Scotland.* Dundee: Scottish Commission for the Regulation of Care.

Chang F. *et al.* (2005). 'The effects of a music programme during lunchtime on the problem behaviour of the older residents with dementia at an institution in Taiwan.' *Journal of Clinical Nursing, 19*, 7, 939–948.

Churchill, M., Safaoui, J., McCabe, B. and Baun, M. (1999) 'Using a therapy dog to alleviate the agitation and desocialisation of people with Alzheimer's disease'. *Journal of Psychosocial Nursing and Mental Health Services 37*, 16–22.

Chung, J.C.C. and Lai, C.K.Y. (2002) 'Snoezelen for dementia'. *Cochrane Database of Systematic Reviews: Reviews Issue 4.* Chichester: John Wiley.

Chung, J.C.C. and Lai, C.K.Y. (2008) 'Snoezelen for dementia'. *Cochrane Database of Systematic Reviews: updated review.*

Clare, L., Woods, B., Moniz-Cooke, E. et al. (2003) 'Cognitive rehabilitation and cognitive training interventions targeting memory functioning in early stage dementia and vascular dementia'. *Cochrane Database of Systematic Reviews, Issue 4.*

Clark, D.M. (1983) 'On the induction of depressed mood in the laboratory: evaluation and comparison of the Velten and musical procedure'. *Advances in Behaviour Research and Therapy 5*, 27–49.

Cohen-Mansfield, J. (2000a) 'Use of patient characteristics to determine nonpharmacologic interventions for behavioural and psychological symptoms of dementia'. *International Psychogeriatrics 12*, 1, 373–386.

Cohen-Mansfield, J. (2000b) 'Nonpharmacological management of behavioural problems in persons with dementia: the TREA model'. *Alzheimer Care Quarterly 1*, 22–34.

Cohen-Mansfield, J. (2001) 'Nonpharmacologic interventions for inappropriate behaviors in dementia: A review, summary and critique'. *American Journal of Geriatric Psychiatry 9*, 361–381.

Cohen-Mansfield, J. (2006) 'Pain assessment in non-communicative elderly persons'. *The Clinical Journal of Pain 22*, 6, 569–575.

Cohen-Mansfield, J., Libin, A. and Marx M. (2007) 'Nonpharmacological treatment of agitation: a controlled trial of systematic individualized intervention'. *Journal of Gerontology: Medical Sciences 62A*, 8, 906–918.

Cohen-Mansfield, J. and Lipson, S. (2002) 'Pain in cognitively impaired nursing home residents: How well are physicians diagnosing it'. *Journal of American Geriatric Association 50*, 6, 1039–1044.

Cohen-Mansfield, J., Marx, M. and Rosenthal, A. (1989) 'A description of agitation in a nursing home'. *Journal of Gerontology: Medical Sciences 44*, 3, M77–84.

Cohen-Mansfield J., Thein, K., Dakheel-Ali, M. and Marx, M. (2010) 'The underlying meaning of stimuli: impact of engagement of person with dementia.' *Psychiatry Research, 15* 177, 216–222.

Commission for Healthcare Audit and Inspection (CHAI) (2006) *Living Well in Later Life: A Review of Progress Against the National Service Framework for Older People.* London: Commission for Healthcare Audit and Inspection.

Cummings, J.L., Mega, M., Gray, K., Rosenberg-Thompson, S., Carusi, D.A. and Gornbein, J. (1994) 'The neuropsychiatric inventory: comprehensive assessment of psychopathology in dementia'. *Neurology 44*, 2308–2314.

Cunningham, J. (2005) *Care staff views about telling the absolute truth to people with dementia.* Submitted in part fulfilment of Doctorate in Clinical Psychology. Ridley Building, Newcastle upon Tyne, UK.

Dagnan, D., Grant, F. and McDonnell, A. (2004) 'Understanding challenging behaviour in older people: the development of the Controllability Beliefs Scale'. *Behavioural and Cognitive Psychotherapy 32*, 4, 501–506.

Darwin, C. (1872) *The Expression of the Emotions in Man and Animals.* London: Murray.

Day, K., Carreon, D. and Stump, C. (2000) 'Therapeutic design of environments for people with dementia: A review of the empirical research'. *The Gerontologist 40*, 397–416.

Dean, R., Proudfoot, R. and Lindesay, J. (1993) 'The quality of interactions scale (QUIS): development, reliability and use in the evaluation of two domus units'. *International Journal of Geriatric Society 8*, 10, 819–826.

Dementia Services Development Centre (DSDC) (2008) *Best Practice in Design for People with Dementia.* Stirling: Dementia Services Development Centre, University of Stirling.

Dempsey, O.P. and Moore, H. (2005) 'Psychotropic prescribing for older people in residential care in the UK, are guidelines being followed?' *Primary Care and Community 10*, 1, 13–18.

DePaulo, B.M., Kashy, D.A., Kirkendol, S.E., Wyer, M.M. and Epstein, J.A. (1996) 'Lying in everyday life'. *Journal of Personality and Social Psychology 70*, 979–995.

Dexter- Smith, S. (2010) 'Integrating psychological formulations into older people's services: three years on'. *PSIGE Newsletter 112*, 3–7.

DoH (2001) *National Service Framework for Older People.* London: Department of Health.

DoH (2005) *Everybody's Business: Integrated Health Services for Older People.* London: Department of Health.

DoH (2009) *National Dementia Strategy.* Living well with dementia: A National Dementia Strategy. (www.dh.gov.uk/en/socialcare/deliveringadultsocialcare/olderpeople/National dementiastrategy/index.htm)

Doyle, C., Zapparoni, T., O'Connor, D. and Runci, S. (1997) 'Efficacy of psychological treatments for noisemaking in severe dementia'. *International Psychogeriatrics 9*, 405–422.

Dynes, R. (2009) Improving communication skills – issues 23–26. www.robindynes.co.uk.

Edwards, N. (2004) 'Using Aquariums in Managing Alzheimer's Disease: Influence on Resident Nutrition and Behaviours and Improving Staff Morale'. In: S.F.C.A. Studies (ed.) *People and Animals: A Timeless Relationship.* Glasgow, IAHAIO.

Eells, T., Kendjelic, E. and Lucas, C. (1998) 'What's in a case formulation: development and use of content coding manual'. *Journal of Psychotherapy Practice and Research 7*, 144–153.

Eggermont, L. and Scherder, E. (2006) 'Physical activity and behaviour in dementia: a review of the literature and implications for psychosocial interventions in primary care'. *Dementia: The International Journal of Social Research and Practice 5*, 3, 411–428.

Ehrenfeld, M. (2003) 'Using therapeutic dolls with psychogeriatric patients'. In: C.E. Schaefer (ed.) *Play Therapy with Adults.* New York: John Wiley.

Ekman, P. (1973) 'Cross Cultural Studies of Facial Expression'. In: P. Ekman (ed.) *Darwin and Facial Expressions: A Century of Research in Review.* New York: Academic Press.

Ellingford, J., James, I., Mackenzie, L. and Marsland, L. (2007) 'Using dolls to alter behaviour in patients with dementia'. *Nursing Times 103*, 5, 36–37.

Elvish, R., James, I.A. and Milne, D. (2010) 'Lying in dementia care: an example of a culture that deceives in people's best interests'. *Aging and Mental Health 14*, 3, 255–262.

Expert Consensus Panel for Agitation in Dementia (1998). 'Treatment of agitation in older persons with dementia.' *Postgraduate Medicine 1*, 1–88.

Feil, N. and de Klerk-Rubin, V. (2002) *The Validation Breakthrough: Simple Techniques for Communicating with People with Alzheimer-Type-Dementia.* Health Professions Press.

Finnema E. *et al.* (2005) 'The effect of integrated emotion-oriented care versus usual care on elderly persons with dementia in the nursing home and on nursing assistants: a randomized clinical trial'. *International Journal of Geriatric Psychiatry 20*, 330–343.

Folstein, M., Folstein, S. and. McHugh, P. (1975) 'The mini-mental state. A practical method for grading the cognitive state of patients for the clinician'. *Journal Psychiatric Research 12*, 189–198.

Fopma-Loy, J. (1991) *Predictors of Caregiver Behavior of Formal Caregivers of Institutionalised People with Dementing Illnesses.* Unpublished doctorate dissertation. University School of Nursing, Indiana.

Forbes, D., Forbes, D., Morgan, M. et al. (2008) 'Physical activity programs for persons with dementia'. *Cochrane Database of Systematic Reviews, Issue 3.*

Forbes, D., Culum, I. and Lischka, A. (2009) 'Light therapy for managing cognitive, sleep, functional, behavioural or psychiatric disturbances in dementia'. *Cochrane Database of Systematic Reviews, Issue 4.*

Fossey, J. and James, I.A. (2007) *Evidence-based Approaches for Improving Dementia Care in Care Homes.* London: Alzheimer's Society.

Fossey, J., Ballard, C., Juszczak, E., James, I., Alder, N., Jacoby, R. and Howard, R. (2006) 'Effect of enhanced psychosocial care on antipsychotic use in nursing home residents with severe dementia: cluster randomised trial'. *Bristish Medical Journal 332*, 756–758.

Fraser, F. and James, I. (2008) 'Why does doll therapy improve the well-being of some older adults with dementia?' *PSIGE Newsletter 105*, 55–63.

Gates, G. *et al.* (2008) 'Central auditory dysfunction in older persons with memory impairment or Alzheimer dementia'. *Archives of Otolaryngology and Head and Neck Surgery 134*, 771–777.

Garner, P. (2004) A SPECAL place to keep. *Journal of Dementia Care 12*, 3.

Gauthier, S. Wirth, Y. and Mobius, H. (2005) 'Effects of behavioural syndromes in Alzheimer disease patients'. *International Journal of Geriatric Psychiatry 20*, 459–464.

Gauthier, S., Loft, H. and Cummings, J. (2008) 'Improvements in behavioural symptoms with moderate to severe Alzheimer's disease by memantine: a pooled data analysis'. *International Journal of Geriatric Psychiatry 23*, 537–545.

Godfrey, S. (1994) 'Doll therapy'. *Australian Journal of Ageing 13*, 1, 46.

Gotell. E., Brown, S. and Ekman, S. (2002) 'Caregiver singing and background music in dementia care'. *Western Journal Nursing Research 24*, 2, 195–216.

Gibson, F. (1994) 'What can Reminiscence Contribute to People with Dementia?' In: J. Bornat (ed.) *Reminiscence Reviewed: Evaluations, Achievements, Perspectives* (pp.46–60). Buckingham: Open University Press.

Gibson, S. (2005) 'A personal experience of successful doll therapy'. *Journal of Dementia Care 13*, 3, 22–23.

Gibson, M.C., MacLean, J., Borrie, M. and Geiger, J. (2004) 'Orientation behaviors in residents relocated to a redesigned dementia care unit'. *American Journal of Alzheimer's Disease and Other Dementias 19*, 45–49.

Gill, S.S. (2005) 'Atypical antipsychotic drugs and risk of ischaemic stroke: population based retrospective cohort study'. *British Medical Journal 330*, 445.

Goudie, F. and Stokes, G. (1989) 'Understanding confusion'. *Nursing Times 85*, 35–37.

Greer, K.L., Pustay, K.A., Zaun, T.C. and Coppens, P. (2001) 'A comparison of the effects of toys versus live animals on the communication of patients with dementia of the Alzheimer's type'. *Clinical Gerontologist 24*, 157–182.

Guzman-Garcia, A., James, I.A. and Mukaetova-Ladinska, E. (in press) 'Danzon a Psychomotor intervention: a piolet'. *Dementia: International Journal of Social Research and Practice.*

Health Economic Research Centre (HERC) (2010) *Dementia 2010: The Economic Burden of Dementia and Associated Research Funding in the UK.* A report produced by the Health Economic Research Centre, University of Oxford for the Alzheimer's Research Trust. (www.alzheimers-research.org.uk).

Heyn, P., Abreu, B. and Ottenbacher, K. (2004) 'The effects of exercise training on elderly persons with cognitive impairment and dementia: a meta-analysis'. *Archives of Physical Medicine and Rehabilitation 85*, 1694–1704.

Hirst, J. and Oldknow, H. (2009) 'Rapid access for older people to specialist mental health services'. *Nursing Times 105*, 7, 12–13.

Hogan, D., Maxwell, C., Fung, T. and Ebly, E. (2003) 'Prevalence and potential consequences of benzodiazepine use in senior citizens: Results from the Canadian Study of Health and Aging'. *Canadian Journal of Clinical Pharmacology 10*, 2, 72–77.

Holden, U. and Woods, B. (1982) *Reality Orientation: Psychological Approaches to the Confused Elderly.* Edinburgh: Churchill Livingstone.

Holland, T. (2008) *The Use of Medication in the Treatment of Challenging Behaviour.* Information sheet of The Challenging Behaviour Foundation (www.Challengingbehaviour.org.uk).

Holmes, C. (2009) *Guidelines: managing behaviour problems in patients with dementia (version 1).* Hampshire Partnership NHS Foundation Trust (www. Hampshirepartnership.nhs.uk).

Holmes, C., Hopkins, V. Hensford, C., MacLaughlin, V., Wilkinson, D. and Rosenvinge, H. (2002) 'Lavender oil as a treatment for agitated behaviour in severe dementia: a placebo controlled study'. *International Journal of Geriatric Psychiatry 17*, 4, 305–308.

Holmes, C., Wilkinson, D., Dean, C. *et al.* (2004). 'The efficacy of donepezil in the treatment of neuropsychiatric symptoms in Alzheimer disease'. *Neurology 63*, 214–219.

Holt, F., Birks, T., Thorgrimsen, L. *et al.* (2003) 'Aromatherapy for dementia'. *Cochrane Database of Systematic Reviews, Issue 3* (last updated 2009).

Hopman-Rock, M., Staats, P., Erwin, C. and Droes, R.-M. (1999) 'The effects of a psychomotor activation programme for use in groups of cognitively impaired people in homes for the elderly'. *International Journal of Geriatric Psychiatry 14*, 8, 633–642.

Howard, R., Ballard, C., O'Brien, J. and Burns, A. (2001) 'Guidelines for the management of agitation in dementia'. *International Journal Geriatric Psychiatry 16*, 714–717.

Hughes, C., Bergh, L. and Danziger, W. (1982) 'A new clinical scale for the staging of dementia'. *British Journal of Psychiatry 140*, 566–572.

Hulme, C. Wright, J., Crocker, T., *et al.* (2010) 'Non-pharmacological approaches for dementia that informal carers might try to access: a systematic review'. *International Journal of Geriatric Psychiatry 25*, 756–763.

Hurley A., Volicer, B. and Hanrahan, P. (2001) 'Assessment of discomfort in advanced Alzheimer's patients.' *Research Nursing Health, 15*, 369–377.

Jackson, G. (2005) 'Anti-psychotic drug use for people with dementia in care homes'. *Journal of Dementia Care Jul–Aug*, 28–30.

James, I.A. (1999) 'Using a cognitive rationale to conceptualise anxiety in people with dementia'. *Behavioural and Cognitive Psychotherapy 27*, 4, 345–351.

James, I.A. (2001) 'The anger triad and its use with people with severe dementia'. *Psychology Special Interest Group for Older People (PSIGE) Newsletter, BPS 76*, 45–47.

James, I.A. (2010) *Cognitive Behavioural Therapy with Older People: Interventions for Those with and Without Dementia.* London: Jessica Kingsley.

James, I.A., Powell, I. and Kendell, K. (2001) 'Cognitive therapy for carers: Distinguishing fact from fiction'. *Journal of Dementia Care 9*, 6, 24–26.

James, I.A. and Sabin, N. (2002) 'Safety seeking behaviours: conceptualising a person's reaction to the experience of cognitive confusion'. *Dementia: The International Journal of Social Research and Practice 1*, 1, 37–46.

James, I.A., Postma, K. and Mackenzie, L. (2003a) 'Using an IPT conceptualisation to treat a depressed person with dementia'. *Behaviour and Cognitive Psychotherapy, 31,* 4.

James, I.A., Powell, I. and Kendell, K. (2003b) 'The castle and the know-it-all – access to the inner circle'. *Journal of Dementia Care 11,* 4, 24–26.

James, I.A., Powell, I. and Kendell, K. (2003c) 'A cognitive perspective on training in care homes'. *Journal of Dementia Care 11,* 3, 22–24.

James, I.A., Powell, I., Smith, T. and Fairbairn, A. (2003d) 'Lying to residents: can the truth sometimes be unhelpful for people with dementia?' *PSIGE Newsletter, BPS 82,* 26–28.

James, I., Reichelt, F., Morse, R., Mackenzie, L. and Mukaetova-Ladinska, E. (2005) 'The therapeutic use of dolls in dementia care'. *Journal of Dementia Care 13,* 3, 19–21.

James, I., Mackenzie, L. and Mukaetova-Ladinska, E. (2006a) 'Doll use in care homes for people with dementia'. *International Journal of Geriatric Psychiatry 21,* 11, 1044–1051.

James, I.A., Mackenzie, L., Stephenson, M. and Roe, P. (2006b) 'Dealing with Challenging Behaviour through an Analysis of Need: the Colombo Approach'. In: M. Marshall (ed.) *On the Move: Walking not Wandering.* London: Hawker Press.

James, I.A., Mukaetova-Ladinska, E., Reichelt, F., *et al.* (2006c) 'Diagnosing Asperger's in the elderly'. *International Journal of Geriatric Psychiatry 21,* 951–960.

James, I.A., Wood-Mitchell, A., Waterworth, A.M., Mackenzie, L. and Cunningham, J. (2006d) 'Lying to people with dementia: developing ethical guidelines for care settings'. *International Journal of Geriatric Psychiatry 21,* 800–801.

James, I.A., Carlson-Mitchell, P., Ellingford, J. and Mackenzie, L. (2007) 'Promoting attitude change: staff training programme on continence care'. *PSIGE Newsletter 97,* 11–16.

James, I.A. and Stephenson, M. (2007) Behaviour that challenges us: the Newcastle support model. *Journal of Dementia Care 15,* 5, 19–22.

James, I.A., Morse, R. and Howarth, A. (2010) 'The science and art of asking questions in cognitive therapy'. *Behavioural and Cognitive Psychotherapy 38,* 1, 83–94.

Johnson, C., Knight, C. and Stewart, I. (2008) 'Just how challenging can older people be? Part 1: Selecting the appropriate tool for measuring aggression within services'. *PSIGE Newsletter 103,* 46–64.

Judd, S., Marshall, M. and Phippen, P. (1997) *Design for Dementia.* London: Hawker.

Kaufer, D.I., Cummings, J.L. and Christine, D., *et al.* (1998) 'Assessing the impact of neuropsychiatric symptoms in Alzheimer's disease: the Neuropsychiatric Inventory Caregiver Distress Scale'. *Journal of the American Geriatrics Society 46,* 210–215.

Keefe. F. and Block, A. (1982) 'Development of an observation method for assessing pain behaviour in chronic low back pain patients.' *Behaviour therapy, 13,* 363–375.

Kipling, T., Bailey, M. and Charlesworth, G. (1999) 'The feasibility of a cognitive behavioural therapy group for men with mild/moderate cognitive impairment'. *Behavioural and Cognitive Psychotherapy 27,* 189–193.

Kitwood, T. (1997) *Dementia Reconsidered.* Buckingham: Open University Press.

Kitwood, T. and Bredin, K. (1992) 'Towards a theory of dementia care: personhood and wellbeing'. *Ageing and Society 12,* 269–287.

Killick, J. and Allan, K. (1999) 'The arts in dementia care: tapping a rich resource'. *Journal of Dementia Care 7,* 35–38.

King, A.C., Oman, R.F., Brassington, G.S., Bliwise, D.L. and Haskell, W.L. (1997) 'Moderate-intensity exercise and self-rated quality of sleep in older adults: a randomized controlled trial'. *JAMA 277,* 1, 32–37.

Knapp, M., Thorgrimsen, L., Patel, A., Spector, A., Hallam, A., Woods, B. and Orrell, M. (2006) 'Cognitive stimulation therapy for people with dementia: cost-effectiveness analysis'. *British Journal of Psychiatry 188,* 574–580.

Koder, D.A. (1998) 'Treatment of anxiety in the cognitively impaired elderly: can cognitive behaviour therapy help?' *International Psychogeriatrics 10,* 2, 173–182.

Kovach, C., Weissman, D., Griffie, J. *et al.* (1999) 'Assessment and treatment of discomfort for people in late-stage dementia'. *Journal of Pain Symptoms Management 18,* 412–419.

Kunik, M., Martinez, M., Snow, A. *et al.* (2003) 'Determinants of behavioural symptoms in dementia patients'. *Clinical Gerontology 26,* 3, 83–89.

Lantz, M., Giambianco, V. and Buchalter, E. (1996) 'A ten-year review of the effect of OBRA 87 on psychotropic prescribing practices in an academic nursing home'. *Psychiatric Services 47*, 951–957.

Lee, P.E., Gill, S.S., Freedman, M., Bronskill, S.E., Hillmer, M.P. and Rochon, P.A. (2004) 'Atypical antipsychotic drugs in the treatment of behavioural and psychological symptoms of dementia: systematic review'. *British Medical Journal 329*, 75–78.

Levin, H.S., High, W.M., Goethe, K.E., Sisson, R.A., Overall, J.E., Rhoades, H.M., Eisenberg, H.M., Kalisky, Z. and Gary, H.E. (1987) 'The neurobehavioural rating scale: assessment of the behavioural sequelae of head injury by the clinician'. *Journal of Neurology, Neurosurgery and Psychiatry 50*, 2,183–193.

Levy-Storms, L. (2008) 'Therapeutic communication training in long-term care institutions: recommendations for future research'. *Patient Education and Counseling 73*, 8–21.

Libin, A. and Cohen-Mansfield, J. (2004) 'Therapeutic Robocat for nursing home residents with dementia: Preliminary inquiry'. *American Journal of Alzheimer's Disease and Other Dementias 19*, 2, 111–116.

Livingston, G., Johnston, K., Katona, C., Paton, J. and Lyketsos, C. (2005) 'Systematic review of psychological approaches to the management of neuropsychiatric symptoms of dementia'. *American Journal of Psychiatry 162*, 11, 1996–2021.

Lord, T. and Garner, E. (1993) 'Effects of music on Alzheimer patients'. *Perceptual and Motor Skills 76*, 451–455.

Lyketsos, C., Lopez, O. and Jones, B. (2002) 'Prevalence of neuropsychiatric symptoms in dementia and mild cognitive impairment: results from the cardiovascular health study'. *JAMA 288*, 1475–1483.

McGilton, K.S. *et al.* (2009) 'A systematic review of the effectiveness of communication interventions for health care providers caring for patients in residential care settings'. *Worldviews Evidence Based Nursing 6*, 3, 149–159.

McGrath, A.M. and Jackson, G.A. (1996) 'A survey of anti-psychotic drug use in nursing homes in Glasgow'. *British Medical Journal 312*, 611–612.

McShane, R., Keene, J., Gedling, K., Fairburn, C., Jacoby, R. and Hope, T. (1997) 'Do anti-psychotic drugs hasten cognitive decline in dementia? Prospective study with necropsy follow up'. *British Medical Journal 314*, 266–270.

McShane, R., Areosa Sastre, A. and Minakaran, N. (2006) 'Memantine for dementia'. *Cochrane Database of Systematic Reviews. Issue 2.*

Mackenzie, L. (2004) *Assessing the Toileting Habits of Staff as a Method of Improving Toileting Regimes in Care.* National Conference of Dementia Care, Harrogate, November 2004.

Mackenzie, L. (2008) *Newcastle Approach to Treatment of CB.* Presentation at National Dementia Congress, Hawker Press (Bournemouth, UK, Nov.)

Mackenzie, L., James, I.A., Morse, R, Mukaetova-Ladinska, E. and Reichelt, F.K. (2006) 'A pilot study on the use of dolls for people with dementia'. *Age and Ageing 35*, 4, 441–444.

Mackenzie, L., Wood-Mitchell, A. and James, I.A. (2007) 'Guidelines on the use of dolls in care settings'. *Journal of Dementia Care 15*, 1, 26–27.

Mahoney, F. and Barthel, D. (1965) 'Functional evaluation: The Barthel Index'. *Maryland State Medical Journal 14*, 61–65.

Makin, S. (2009) *Formulation-driven Approaches to Agitated Behaviour.* Dissertation for Doctorate in Clinical Psychology, Newcastle University, UK.

Maslow, A. (1943) 'Theory of human motivation'. *Psychosomatic Medicine 5*, 85–92.

Mayers, K. (2003) 'Play Therapy for Individuals with Dementia'. In: C.E. Schaefer (ed.) *Play Therapy with Adults.* New York: John Wiley and Sons.

Meehan, K.M., Wang, H., David, S.R., Nisivoccia, J.R., Jones, B. et al. (2002) 'Comparison of rapidly acting intra-muscular olanzapine, lorazepam and placebo: a double blind randomised study in acutely agitated patients with dementia'. *Neuropsychopharmacology 26*, 494–594

Mental Capacity Act (2005) legislation.gov.uk/ukpga/2005/9/contents.

Miller M. (2008) *Clinician's Guide to Interpersonal Psychotherapy in Late Life: Helping Cognitively Impaired or Depressed Elders and Their Caregivers.* New York: Oxford University Press.

Miller, M. and Reynolds, C.F. (2002) ,Interpersonal Psychotherapy'. In: J. Hepple, J. Pearce and P. Wilkinson (eds). *Psychological Therapies with Older People*. London: Bruner-Routledge.

Miller, M. and Reynolds, C. (2007) 'Expanding the usefulness of interpersonal psychotherapy (IPT) for depressed elders with comorbid cognitive impairment'. *International Journal of Geriatric Psychiatry 11*, 97–102.

Mioshi, E., Dawson, K., Mitchell, J., *et al.* (2006) 'The Addenbrooke's Cognitive Examination revised (ACE-R). A brief cognitive test battery for dementia screening'. *International Journal of Geriatric Psychiatry 2*, 11, 1078–1085.

Moniz-Cook, E. Woods, R. and Gardiner E. (2000) 'Staff factors associated with perception of behaviour as challenging in residential and nursing homes'. *Aging and Mental Health 4*, 48–55.

Moniz-Cook, E., Woods, R. and Richards, K. (2001a) 'Functional analysis of challenging behaviour in dementia: the role of superstition'. *International Journal of Geriatric Psychiatry 16*, 45–56.

Moniz-Cook, E., Woods, R., Gardiner, E., Silver, M. and Agar, S. (2001b) 'The Challenging Behaviour Scale (CBS): development of a scale for staff caring for older people in residential and nursing homes'. *British Journal of Clinical Psychology 40*, 3, 309–322.

Moniz-Cook, E., Vernooij-Dassen, M., Woods, R. et al. (2008a) 'A European consensus on outcome measures for psychological intervention research in dementia'. *Aging and Mental Health 12*, 1, 14–29.

Moniz-Cook, E., De Vught, M., Verhey, F. and James, I. (2008b) 'Functional analysis-based interventions for challenging behaviour in dementia'. *Cochrane Database of Systematic Reviews, Issue 1*. Art. No.: CD006929. DOI: 10.1002/14651858.CD006929.

Moniz-Cook *et al.* (2008c) 'Can training community mental health nurses to support family carers reduce behavioural problems in dementia? An exploratory pragmatic randomised controlled trial.' *International Journal of Geriatric Psychiatry, 23*, 2, 185–191.

Moniz-Cook, E., Walker, A., De Vught, M., Verhey, F. and James, I. (in press) 'Functional analysis based interventions for challenging behaviour in dementia – (Cochrane Review)'. *Cochrane Database of Systematic Reviews*.

Montgomery, P. and Dennis, J. (2002) 'Physical exercise for sleep problems in adults aged 60+'. *Cochrane Database of Systematic Reviews: Reviews Issue 4*. Chichester: John Wiley.

Moore, D. (2001) '"It's like a gold medal and it's mine" – dolls in dementia care'. *Journal of Dementia Care 9*, 6, 20–22.

Moriaty, J., Treadgold, M. and Grennan, S. (2003) 'Activating potential for communication through all the senses'. *Dementia 2*, 2.

Mottram, P. (2003) 'Art therapy with clients who have dementia'. *Dementia 2*, 272–277.

NAO (2007) 'Improving services and support for people with dementia'. HC 604 (July).

Neal, M. and Barton Wright, P. (2003) 'Validation therapy for dementia'. *Cochrane Database of Systematic Reviews: Reviews Issue 3*. Chichester: John Wiley.

Neville, C. and Bryne, G. (2001) 'Literature review: behaviour rating scales for older people with dementia: which is the best for use by nurses?' *Australasian Journal Ageing 20*, 166–172.

NICE (2004) 'Depression: management of depression in primary and secondary care – Clinical guideline 23' (www.nice.org.uk/CG023).

NICE (2006) 'Dementia: supporting people with dementia and their carers'. *NICE-SCIE Clinical Guideline 42*. London: DoH.

Orrell, M. and Woods, R. (1996) 'Tacrine and psychological therapies – no contest'. *International Journal of Geriatric Psychiatry 11*, 189–192.

Perrin, T. and May, H. (2000) *Wellbeing in Dementia: An Occupational Approach for Therapists and Carers*. Churchill Livingstone: London.

Porteinsson, A.P., *et al.* (2001) 'Placebo-controlled study of divalproex sodium for agitation in dementia'. *American Journal of Geriatric Psychiatry 9*, 58–66.

Pollock, B., *et al.* (2002) 'Comparison of citalopram, perphenazine, and placebo for the acute treatment of psychosis and behavioural disturbances in hospitalised demented patients'. *American Journal of Psychiatry 159*, 460–465.

Price J., Hermans D. and Grimley E. (2001) *Subjective Barriers to Prevent Wandering of Cognitively Impaired People.* The Cochrane Database of Systematic Reviews Chichester: Wiley (updated 2009).

Quynh-anh, N. and Paton, C. (2008) 'The use of aromatherapy to treat behaviour problems in dementia'. *International Journal of Geriatric Psychiatry 27,* 4, 337–346.

Renaud, D., Mulin, E., Mallea, P. and Robert, P. (2010) 'Measurement of neuropsychiatric symptoms in clinical trials targeting Alzheimer's disease and related disorders.' *Pharmaceuticals, 3,* 2387–2397.

Richeson, N. (2003) 'Effects of animal assisted therapy on agitated behaviours and social interactions of older adults with dementia.' *American Journal of Alzheimers Disease and Other Dementias, 18,* 6, 353–358.

Romero, B., and Wenz, M. (2001) 'Self-maintenance therapy in Alzheimer's disease'. *Neuropsychological Rehabilitation 11,* 333–355.

Schaie, K.W. (2008) 'A Lifespan Developmental Perspective of Psychological Ageing'. In: K. Laidlaw and B. Knight (eds). *Handbook of Emotional Disorders in Later Life: Assessment and Treatment* (pp.3–32). Oxford: Oxford University Press.

Schneider, L., Dagerman, K. and Insel, P. (2005) 'Risk of death with atypical antipsychotic drug treatment for dementia: meta-analysis of randomised placebo-controlled trials'. JAMA *294,* 1934–1943.

Schols, J., Crebolder, H. and van Weel, C. (2004) 'Nursing home and nursing home physician: the Dutch experience'. *Journal of the American Medical Directors Association 5,* 3, 207–212.

Schrijnemaekers, V., Rossum, E.,van Heusden, M. *et al.* (2002) 'Compliance in a randomised controlled trial: the implementation of emotion-orientated care in psycho-geriatric facilities'. *Journal of Advanced Nursing 39,* 2, 182–189.

Scott, B. (2009) *A Staff Survey of Helpful Aspects of Interventions for Individuals Whose Behaviour Challenges Services.* Dissertation (SSRP) for Doctorate in Clinical Psychology, Newcastle University, UK.

Scottish Government (2010) *Scotland's National Dementia Strategy.* Edinburgh: The Scottish Government, St Andrew's House.

Sells, D. and Shirley, L. (2010) 'Person centred risk management: the traffic light approach'. *Journal of Dementia Care 18,* 5, 21–23.

Shankar, K., Walker, M., Frost, D. and Orrell, M. (1999) 'The development of a valid and reliable scale for rating anxiety in dementia (RAID)'. *Aging and Mental Health 3,* 39–49.

Sherrat, K., Thornton, A. and Hatton, C. (2004) 'Music interventions for people with dementia: a review of the literature'. *Journal Mental Health and Aging 8,* 1, 3–12.

Shirley, L.J. (2005) 'The development of a tool to measure attributional processes in dementia care settings'. *Clinical Psychology Forum 154,* 21–24.

SIGN Scottish Intercollegiate Guidelines Network (1998) *Interventions in the Management of Behavioural and Psychological Aspects of Dementia.* SIGN: Edinburgh.

Singh, N., Stavrinos, T.M., Scarbek, Y., Galambos, G., *et al.* (2005) 'A randomized controlled trial of high versus low intensity weight training versus general practitioner care for clinical depression in older adults'. *Journal of Gerontology (A) Biological and Medical Science 60,* 768–776.

Sink, K.M., Holden, F.H. and Yaffe, K. (2005) 'Pharmacological treatment of neuropsychiatric symptoms of dementia: A review of the evidence'. *Journal of the American Medical Association 293,* 5, 596–608.

Sival, R.C., Hathmans, P.M., Jansen, P.A., Duursma, S.A. and Eikellenboom, P. (2002) 'Sodium valproate in the treatment of aggressive behaviour in patients with dementia: A randomise placebo controlled clinical trial'. *International Journal of Geriatric Psychiatry 17,* 579–585.

Slater, E. and Glazer, W. (1995) 'Use of OBRA-87 guidelines for prescribing neuroleptics in a VA nursing home'. *Psychiatric Services 46,* 119–121.

Sloane, P., Mitchell, C., Preisser, J. *et al.* (1998) 'Environmental correlates of resident agitation in Alzheimer's disease special care units'. *Journal of American Geriatric Society 46,* 862–869.

Smith, K., Milburn, M. and Mackenzie, L. (2008) 'Poor command of English language: a problem in care home? If so, what can be done'. *Journal of Dementia Care 16*, 6, 37–39.

Spector, A, Orrell, M., Davies, S. and Woods, R.T. (2002a) 'Reality Orientation for Dementia' (Cochrane review). In: *The Cochrane Library*. Update Software, issue 2: Oxford.

Spector, A., Thorgrimsen, L., Woods, B., Royan, L., Davies, S., Butterworth, M. and Orrell, M. (2003) 'Efficacy of an evidence-based cognitive stimulation programme for people with dementia: randomised controlled trial'. *British Journal of Psychiatry 183*, 248–254.

Spector, A., Thorgrimsen, L., Woods, B. and Orrell, M. (2006) *Making a Difference: An Evidence-based Group Programme to Offer Cognitive Stimulation Therapy (CST) to People with Dementia*. London: Hawker Publications.

Spira, A. and Edelstein, B. (2006) 'Behavioral interventions for agitation in older adults with dementia: an evaluative review'. *International Psychogeriatrics 18*, 2, 195–225.

Steinberg, M. and Lyketsos, C. (2005) 'Pharmacological treatment of neuropsychiatric symptoms of dementia'. *Journal of American Medical Association 293*, 18, 2211–2212.

Stokes, G. (2001) *Challenging Behaviour in Dementia: A Person-centred Approach*. Bicester, UK: Speechmark.

Stolee, P., Hillier, L., Esbaugh, J., Bol, N., McKellar, L. and Gauthier, N. (2005). 'Instruments for the assessment of pain in older people with cognitive impairment.' *Journal of American Geriatric Society, 53*, 319–326.

Sunderland T., Hill, J., Lawlor, B. and Molchan, S. (1988) *Psychopharmacological Bulletin, 24*, 4, 747–753.

Suzuki, M., Kanamori, M., Watanabe, M., Nagasawa, S., Kojima, E., Ooshiro, H. and Nakahara, D. (2004) 'Behavioral and endocrinological evaluation of music therapy for elderly patients with dementia'. *Nursing and Health Sciences 6*, 11–18.

Tariot, P.N., Schneider, L.S., Mintzer, J., Cutler, A., Cunningham, M., *et al.* (2001) 'Safety and tolerability of divalproex sodium in the treatment of signs and symptoms of mania in elderly patients with dementia: results of a double blind, placebo controlled trial'. *Current Theories in Research and Clinical Experimentation 62*, 51–67.

Taylor, D. (2010) 'Antipsychotic polypharmacy – confusion reigns'. *The Psychiatrist (RCPsych) 34*, 41–43.

Teri, L. and Gallagher-Thompson, D. (1991) 'Cognitive-behavioural interventions for treatment of depression in Alzheimer's patients'. *Gerontologist 31*, 3, 413–416.

Teri L., Logsdon, R.G., Uomoto, J., McCurry, S.M. (1997) 'Behavioural treatment of depression in dementia patients: a controlled clinical trial'. *Journal of Gerontology: Psychological Sciences 52B*, 4 159–166.

Thompson, C., Brodaty, H., Trollor, J. and Sachdev, P. (2010) 'Behavioural and psychological symptoms associated with dementia and dementia subtype and severity'. *International Psychogeriatrics 22*, 2, 300–305.

Thwaites, S. and Sara, A. (2010) 'Tailor made cognitive stimulation'. *Journal of Dementia Care 18*, 5, 19–20.

Threadgold, M. (2002) 'Sonas aPc – a new lease of life for some'. *Signpost 7*, 35–36.

Thorgrimsen, L., Spector, A., Wiles, A., *et al.* (2003) 'Aromatherapy for dementia'. *Cochrane Database of Systematic Reviews, Issue 3*.

Toseland, R.W., Diehl, M., Freeman, K., Manzaneres, T., Naleppa, M. and McCallion, P. (1997) 'The impact of validation group therapy on nursing home residents with dementia'. *Journal of Applied Gerontology 16*, 31–50.

Trinh, N., Hoblyn, J., Mohanty, S. and Yaffe. K. (2003) 'Efficacy of cholinesterase inhibitors in the treatment of neuropsychiatric symptoms and functional impairment in Alzheimer disease: a meta-analysis'. *JAMA 289*, 210–216.

van Weert, J., van Dulmen, A., Spreeuwenberg, P., Ribbe, M. and Bensing, J. (2005) 'Effects of snoezelen, integrated in 24h dementia care, on nurse–patient communication during morning care'. *Patient Education and Counseling 58*, 312–326.

van Weert, J., Janssen, B., van Dulmen, A., Spreeuwenberg, P., Ribbe, M. and Bensing, J. (2006) 'Nursing assistants' behaviour during morning care: effects of the implementation of snoezelen, integrated in 24 hr dementia care'. *Journal of Advanced Nursing 53*, 656–668.

Vasse, E., Vernooij-Dassen, M., Spijker, A. Rikket, M.O. and Koopmans, R. (2010) 'A systematic review of communication strategies for people with dementia in residential and nursing homes'. *International Psychogeriatrics 22*, 2, 189–200.

Verkaik, R., van Weert, J. and Francke, A. (2005) 'The effects of psychosocial methods on depressed, aggressive and apathetic behaviours of people with dementia: a systematic review'. *International Journal of Geriatric Psychiatry 20*, 301–314.

Vernooij-Dassen, M., Vasse, E., Zuidema, S., *et al.* (2010) 'Psychosocial interventions for dementia patients in long-term care'. *International Psychogeriatrics 22*, 7, 1121–1128.

Vink, A.C. and Birks, J.S. (2003, 2009) 'Music therapy for people with dementia'. *The Cochrane Database Reviews.* The Cochrane Database of Systematic Reviews.

Volicer, L. and Hurley, A. (2003) 'Management of behavioural symptoms in progressive degenerative dementias'. *Journal of Gerontology 58A*, 9, 837–845.

Vrij, A. (2000) 'The Social Psychology of Lying and Detecting Deceit'. In: A. Vrij (ed.) *Detecting Lies and Deceit: The Psychology of Lying and the Implications for Professional Practice* (pp.1–17). Chichester: John Wiley.

Wagner, A., Zhang, F., Soumerai, S. *et al.* (2004) 'Benzodiazepine use and hip fractures in the elderly: who is at greatest risk?' *Archives of Internal Medicine 164*, 14, 1567–1572.

Warner, J., Butler, R. and Wuntakal, B. (2006) 'Dementia'. *British Medical Journal Clinical Evidence 12*, 1361–1390.

Waterworth, A, James, I.A., Meyer, T. and Lee, D. (in press) 'Can a lie be therapeutic? The views of people with dementia'. *Aging and Mental Health.*

Wilkinson, N., Srikumar, S., Shaw, K. and Orrell, M. (1998) 'Drama and movement therapy in dementia: a pilot study'. *Arts in Psychotherapy 25*, 3, 195–201.

Wilson, B.A., Evan, J., Alderman, N., Burgess, P. and Emslie, H. (1997) 'Behavioural Assessment of the Dysexecutive Syndrome'. In: P. Rabbit (ed.) *Methodology of Frontal and Executive Function* (pp.239–250). Hove: Psychology Press.

Woods B., Spector A., Orrell M. and Aguirre E. (2009) *Cognitive Stimulation for People with Dementia (Review)* The Cochrane Database of Systematic Reviews Chichester: Wiley

Winstead-Fry, P. and Kijek, J. (1999) 'An integrative review and meta-analysis of therapeutic touch research'. *Alternative Therapies in Health and Medicine 5*, 58–67.

Woods, B., Spector, A., Prendergast, L. and Orrell, M. (2005a) 'Cognitive stimulation to improve cognitive functioning in people with dementia'. *Cochrane Database of Systematic Reviews, Issue 4.*

Woods, B., Spector, A., Jones, C., Orrell, M. and Davies., S. (2005b) 'Reminiscence therapy for dementia'. *Cochrane Database of Systematic Reviews: Reviews Issue 2.* Chichester: John Wiley.

Wood-Mitchell, A., Cunningham, J., Mackenzie, L. and James, I. (2007a) 'Can a lie ever be therapeutic? The debate continues'. *Journal of Dementia Care 15*, 2, 24–28.

Wood-Mitchell, A., James, I.A., Waterworth, A. and Swann, A. (2008) 'Factors influencing the prescribing of medications by old age psychiatrists for behavioural and psychological symptoms of dementia: a qualitative study'. *Age and Ageing 3*, 1–6.

Wood-Mitchell, A., Waterworth, A., Stephenson, M. and James, I. (2006) 'Lying to people with dementia: sparking the debate'. *Journal of Dementia Care 14*, 6, 30–31.

Wood-Mitchell, A., Mackenzie, L., Stephenson, M. and James, I.A. (2007b) 'Treating challenging behaviour in care settings: audit of a community service using the neuropsychiatric inventory'. *PSIGE Newsletter, British Psychological Society 101*, 19–23.

Zeisel, J., Silverstein, N., Hyde, J., *et al.* (2003) 'Environmental correlates to behavioural health outcomes in Alzheimer's special care units'. *Gerontologist 43*, 697–711.

Zuidema, S., de Jonghe, J., Verhey, F. and Koopmans, R. (2010) 'Environmental correlates of neuropsychiatric symptoms in nursing home patients with dementia'. *International Journal of Geriatric Psychiatry 25*, 1, 14–22.

Subject Index

Author Index